Rawsome Flex:
Beautifying System of Facial Exercises and Raw Foods

TONYA ZAVASTA

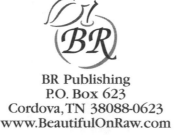

BR Publishing
P.O. Box 623
Cordova, TN 38088-0623
www.BeautifulOnRaw.com

Cover design: John Childress, J&B Childress Portrait Art
Layout: Ken Armstrong
Editors: Sharron K. Carrell, Bradley Harris
Proofreading by Wendy Griffin Anderson and Nick Zavas

Published by:

BR Publishing
P.O. Box 623
Cordova, TN 38088-0623

ISBN-13: 978-0-9742434-7-4

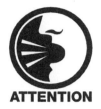

ATTENTION

I recommend that you **do not print** this e-book. There are many pictures here and you'll spend a lot on ink cartridges. No need to print—I designed it as an *e-book*. Read it on your monitor screen. Use it faithfully for 21 days. Then, I *promise* you, you'll know it by heart and won't need a printed copy.

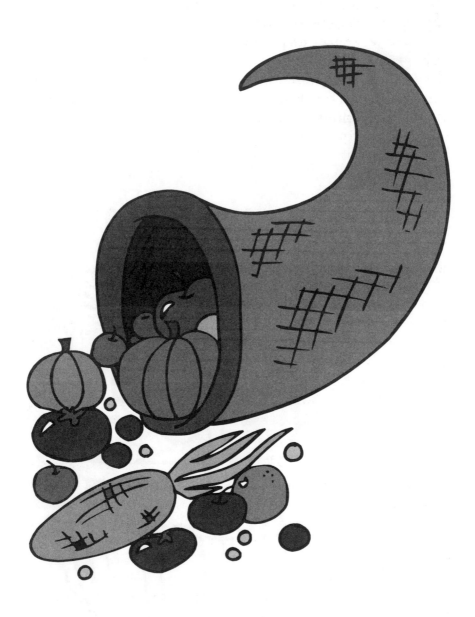

If you're anything like me you're going to want to fly through this introduction and try the exercises right away. That's why my introduction will be short. I placed the most important information *after* the exercises. I understand—what you want to do now is to try the exercises and see if they're worth your time. Mind you, that's like checking your stocks and bonds the very next day after you've bought them. Ain't nothin' happenin' overnight—you have to give them time before judging their performance.

The first three weeks of exercise are crucial to your success. After exercising daily (with maybe a couple of days off) for 21 days, most people will see dramatic results. At that time you *will* want to continue. You *will* find the time and place to do them. Once you see you are being rewarded for your efforts, you'll look forward to your daily regimen. Go ahead and read through all the exercises and try them out.

However, delayed gratification is the name of the game during those first few weeks. You must develop a daily habit. When an action becomes a habit, the probability of continued repetition rises tenfold. But once your habit's there, it's a free ride—your exercising will take very little mental exertion. It saves energy and at the same time relieves us of the burden of decision-making. Do something one way, make a specific choice, and it becomes so much easier to repeat it over and over again.

Researchers say it takes about three weeks to develop a new habit. I see my task as helping and encouraging you day by day during these 21 days. Do not read the entire 21 day program (the section of the e-book which starts after the exercise descriptions) in one sitting. Instead, read it one day at a time over the course of the 21 days. I'm not trying to hide anything from you. Believe me, I want you to succeed as much as you want to look better. Information is useless if you don't act upon it. That is why I introduce something inspirational every day to support you when you need that extra push or encouragement. Each day, I include something intriguing, something to motivate you, something to make you want to work on your face. Do not jeopardize my efforts and your potential progress.

Remember…we hear only what we are ready to hear. If you read the whole e-book in one sitting, you're going to be overwhelmed and you'll likely lose the inspirational element. Information in this e-book is designed to be given to you at intervals, when you're ready to absorb it. The book's structure is not intended to insult your intelligence, but to respect how your brain works. I suspect that only one in a hundred will do as I ask by not reading ahead. This one person will get the most from my e-book.

WARNING

During the first several days new facial lines may appear. Don't panic! These exercises are carefully designed to eliminate wrinkles—not to create new ones. But the bottom line is that if several minutes of facial expressions happen to give you a few new lines, that's simply an indicator of how desperately you need the exercises.

We should not blame the exercises because our skin lacks the elasticity to snap back. Young faces always have this snap-back quality. Pinch a tiny piece of flesh for several seconds, and its youthfulness is shown by how quickly it returns to a plump, smooth appearance. A baby's skin doesn't even notice a crease—it doesn't even last long enough to be called "temporary." The older your skin, the longer that tiny pinch will remain. Try pinching your forearm if you don't want to pinch your face—you'll get the idea either way. That pinch won't leave a permanent mark, I promise.

Do understand that lines etched on our faces are indications of poor muscle tone and greatly aged skin. Every exercise is designed to never create a line on a normally structured face. By "normal" I mean that there are no hanging folds of skin or loose underlying muscles. Exercise itself does not cause problems. Flaccid, unsupported muscles are to blame. Of course, even a young face gets expression lines. But smiles and frowns take decades to become a permanent part of our face. A few days of exercise is *definitely* not going to give you permanent lines. As you keep doing the exercises, the facial muscles will become more and more toned, your skin will gain more elasticity, and those lines will no longer be an issue.

You have reached a crucial moment of decision: Will one extra temporary line stop you from exercising? Or will you concentrate on building the muscle tone that allows you to rejuvenate your skin so it will eventually be able to rebound from the occasional exercise crease?

Now is the time to start an exercise regimen that will help you regain muscle support. These strengthened muscles will firm up your skin. Wrinkles, old creases as well as new, will gradually disappear.

Keep in mind that exercises are just as good for your face as they are for the rest of your body. Nonetheless, every past or present facial exercise expert will remind you: There *is* a period of adjustment. Your face is going through major reorganizing. New muscles are developing. Underlying structure is changing. Your skin is not yet elastic enough and therefore holds creases. As your face develops more elasticity through exercise, it will not maintain these creases. As you continue the exercises, you'll notice that the lines will smooth out.

Those of you on raw foods regimens know that everything real and beneficial for your health has a transition period. And, just like raw foods, facial exercises are not popular because they require patience, persistence, and some adjustment.

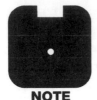

NOTE

If you have any health problems or concerns, I recommend that you discuss these exercises with your health care professional, osteopath, or chiropractor before starting them. Remember, the exercises are there to help and should not cause any pain. If you do experience pain, please stop doing the exercises and refer to your health care practitioner.

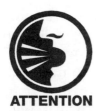

ATTENTION

Take your "Before" pictures now!

To know that you are doing the exercises correctly, you must work your muscles to exhaustion, until you feel they are burning.

Always start your facial exercises by washing your hands and face.

Always finish your facial exercises by applying a good moisturizer.

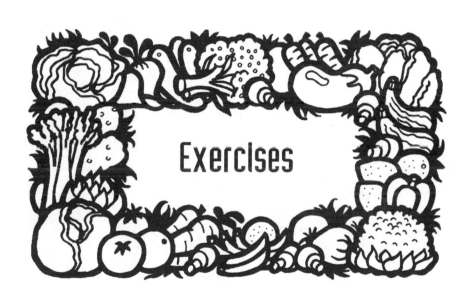

Exercises

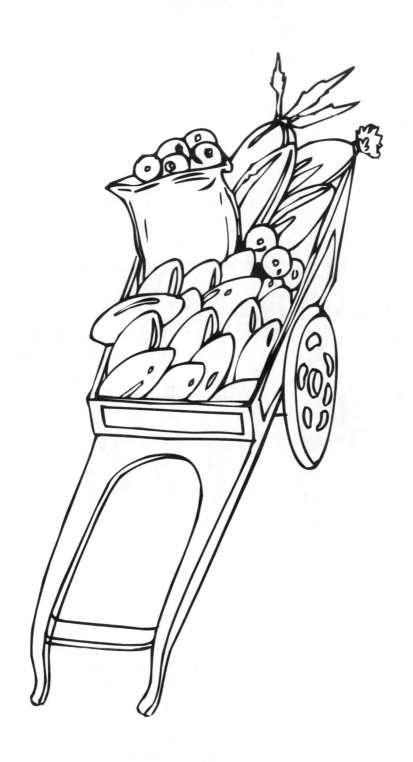

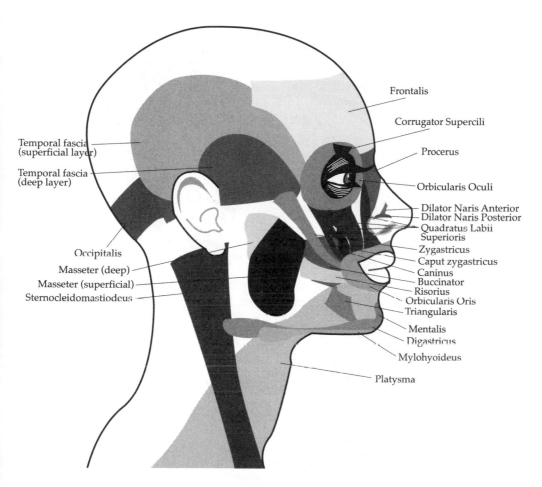

Frontalis

Corrugator Supercili

Procerus

Orbicularis Oculi

Temporal fascia
(superficial layer)

Temporal fascia
(deep layer)

Dilator Naris Anterior
Dilator Naris Posterior
Quadratus Labii
Superioris

Zygastricus
Caput zygastricus
Caninus
Buccinator
Risorius
Orbicularis Oris
Triangularis

Occipitalis

Masseter (deep)

Masseter (superficial)

Sternocleidomastiodeus

Mentalis
Digastricus

Mylohyoideus

Platysma

Facial Muscles Diagram

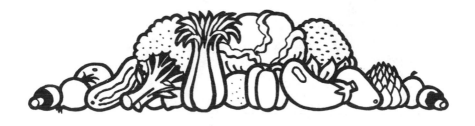

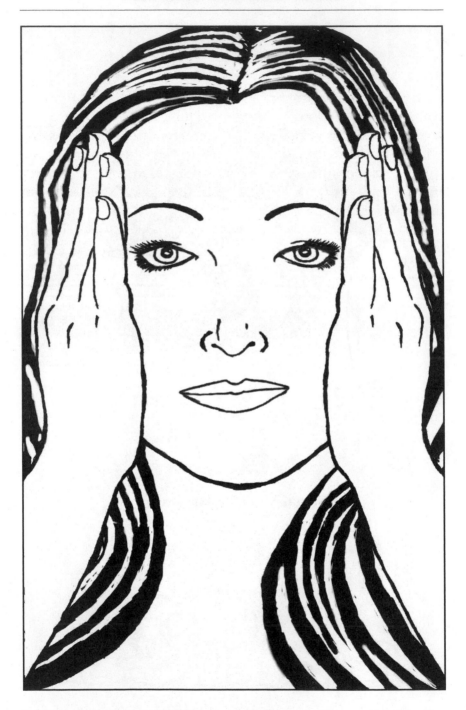

Exercise 1
Warm up

Remember the last time you skinned a chicken breast or trimmed meat (hopefully this was a long time ago before you switched to raw vegan foods)? You saw fascia. Fascia is the whitish colored thin sheets of tissue between the skin and the muscle of the meat. Fascia looks thin, but it is very fibrous and strong. Your body also has fascia. Fascia forms directly under the skin and serves as a strong layer of connective tissue between the skin and the muscles underneath it. It is very important to keep the fascia from becoming glued to the skin or muscles it covers. This exercise will greatly increase circulation in your face and get it ready for these exercises.

1. Sit straight.
2. Place the palms of your hands on both sides of your face, fingers up.
3. Press them tightly to the sides of your face.
4. Move your hands up and down in a small range of motion for a count of 6.
5. Repeat 10 times.

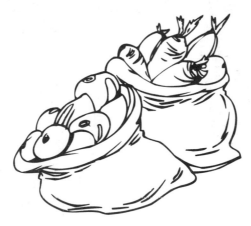

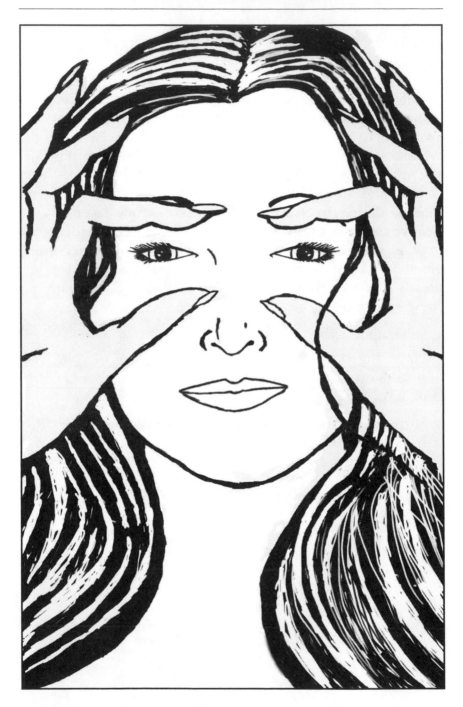

Exercise 2
"Circle the Eye" Flex

This exercise tones the entire eye area by strengthening the *Orbicularis Oculi.*

1. Place your thumbs and index fingers around your eyes. Make an open circle around your eye with your fingers. Open your eyes wide with the help of your fingers.

2. Now close your eyes tightly using your eye muscles.

3. Let your fingers provide gentle resistance that forces the muscles to work hard. Hold the muscles tight for a count of 6.

4. Repeat 10 times.

Normally this muscle action would make lines and creases in the skin. This won't happen because the exercise is designed so that your hands prevent most of the movement in the skin when the muscles contract.

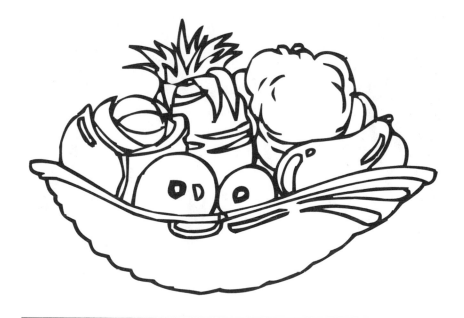

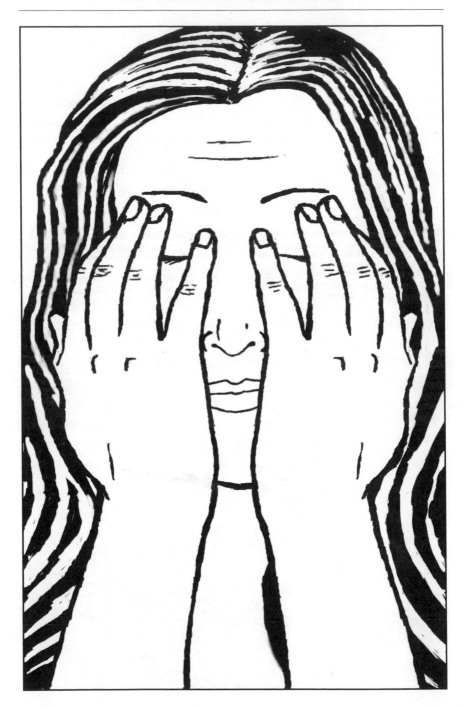

Exercise 3
Upper Lid Flex

Research indicates that the lower eyelids typically stretch over half an inch between the ages of 21 and 60. Whether they quit elongating after 60 or no one even pays attention anymore is unclear. Exercises 2 and 3 can tighten and shorten the muscles around your eyes to a near pre-aging firmness.

1. Place the fingers of each hand just under your eyebrows.
2. Push your fingers up while closing your eyes and stretching your eyelids down.
3. Contract the muscles by closing the eyes, pushing the lids as far down as possible.
4. Hold for a count of 6. Open your eyes and relax the tension of your fingers on your eyebrows after each time
5. Repeat 10 times.

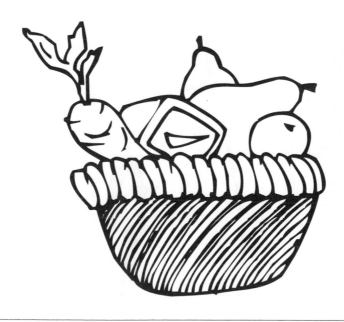

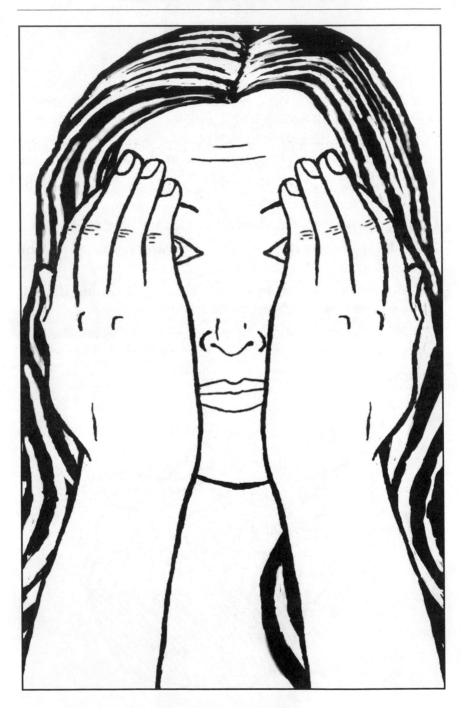

Exercise 4
Brow Raiser

This exercise will build up the *Frontalis Corrugator Supercilii,* making the eyes look larger.

1. Cover your face with your palms. Place the fingers of each hand just above your eyebrows.

2. Apply downward pressure with all of your fingers to hold your forehead firmly in place.

3. Raise your eyebrows as if you are surprised.

4. Hold for a count of 6.

5. Repeat 10 times.

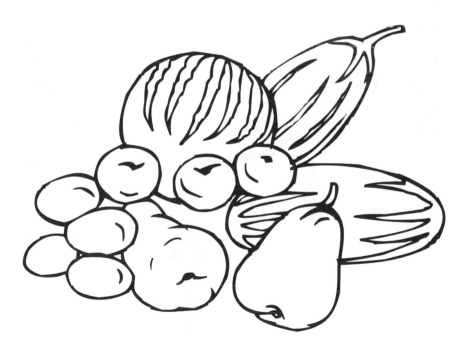

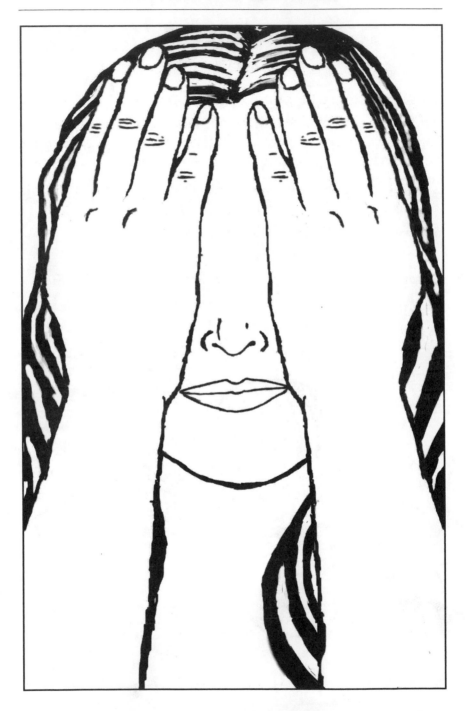

Exercise 5
Palm Suction

This exercise greatly improves circulation in the area around your eyes. It will strengthen the large circular muscle surrounding the eye (*Orbicularis Oculi*) and, when developed, will prevent or eliminate sagginess. If done regularly it will remove eye bags and, at the same time, will plump the area around the eyes—reducing or eliminating "sunken eyes" and "dark circles."

1. Cup your palms over your closed eyes. The palm of each hand will work as a cup pressed tightly against the bony ridges around your eye, but without pressing on the eyes themselves.

2. Without lifting your hands from your skin, create a suction or pumping motion. push and slightly release the pressure. Repeat 10 times.

3. While you are at it, you might want to alternate with another massage technique: keep your hand cupped over your eyes and rotate the wrist slightly, producing a deep tissue massage effect.

This is an excellent exercise, but **DO NOT OVERDO IT!** Be sure you do not bruise the delicate tissue. If you have had detached retinas, you may not want to do this exercise at all.

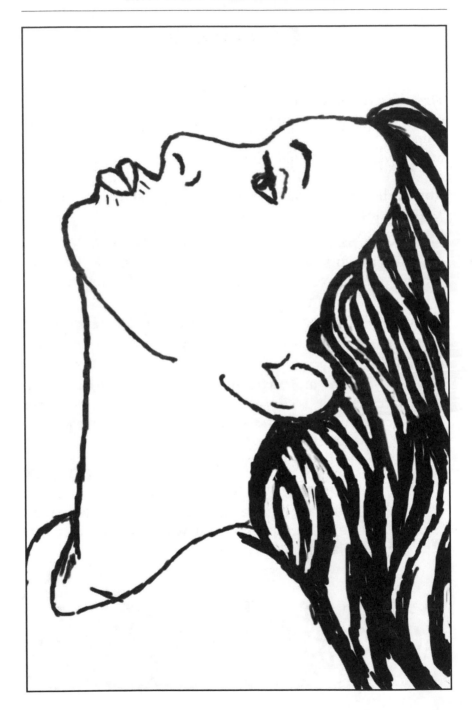

Exercise 6
Kiss the Ceiling

This is a great jaw, neck, and throat firmer.

1. Sit straight. Tilt your head slightly upwards. Pucker your lips together in a kiss and stretch the kiss, as if you are trying to kiss the ceiling.

2. Let each kiss last at least for a count of 6.

3. Repeat 10 times.

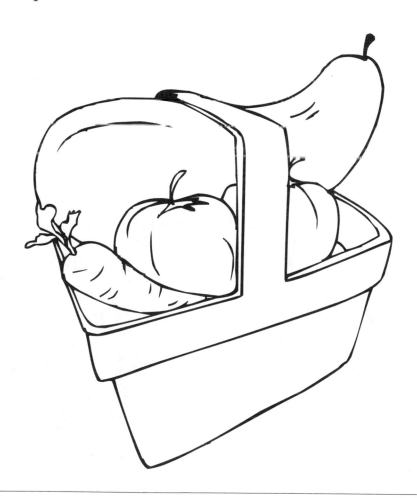

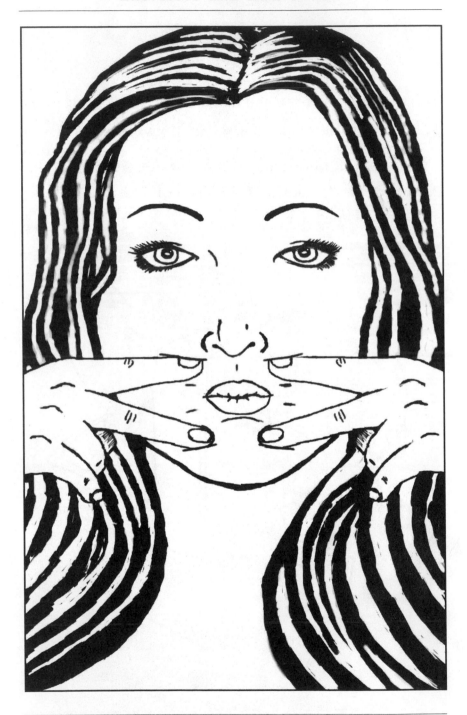

Exercise 7
Kiss Exercise with Resistance

This exercise will build muscles around your mouth, *Orbicularis Oris,* and eliminate wrinkles on the corners of the mouth.

1. Sit straight, tilt the head slightly upward, and purse your lips together.
2. Hold the corners of your mouth by placing the tips of your index fingers flat on the upper edge of your upper lip.
3. Point your fingertips toward each other with your elbows up.
4. Do the same with your middle fingers on the lower edge of your lower lip.
5. Press the fingers away from your mouth to provide counter resistance as you make a kiss.
6. Hold it for a count of 6.
7. Repeat 10 times

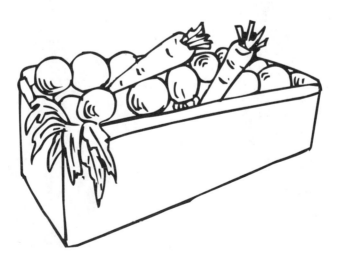

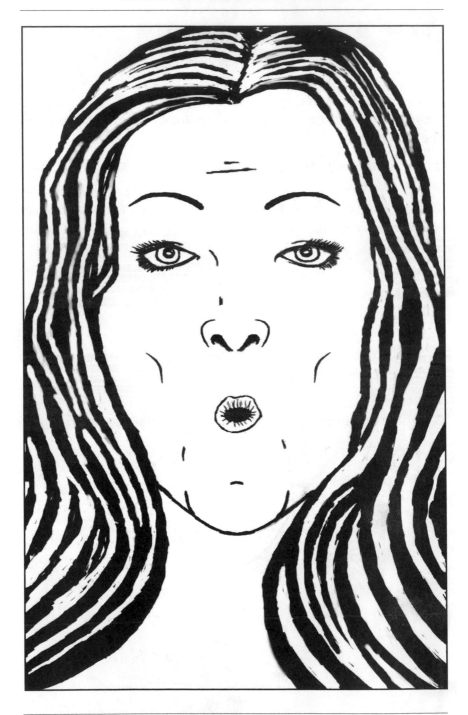

Exercise 8
'O' Exercise

This exercise strengthens all the muscles of your face. It flushes your whole face with new blood. As a result you will feel energized.

1. Sit straight, tilt the head slightly upward.
2. Wrap your upper lip over upper teeth and your lower lip over your lower teeth. Form an 'O' with your lips.
3. Using your lips, make the 'O' smaller, at the same time pressing the lips to the teeth as tightly as possible.
4. Hold the small 'O' for a count of 6. Be sure you feel some burning sensation.
5. Repeat 10 times

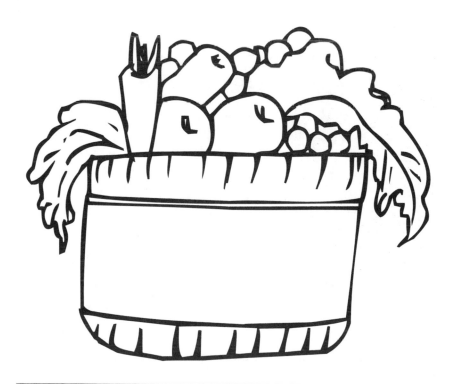

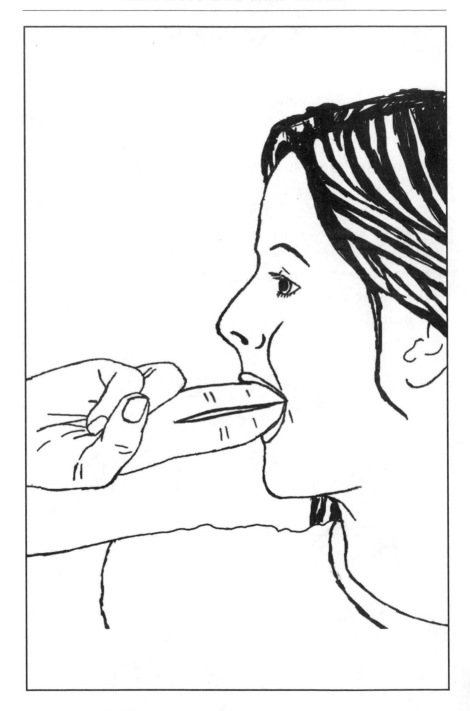

Exercise 9
Squeeze the Fingers

This exercise strengthens every muscle of the lower face. It contributes to fullness of the lips, helps to fill hollows, and lifts sags in the contours of the lower face.

1. Wrap your lips over your teeth. Insert the index and middle fingers of one hand straight between your lips so the fingers are directly under your nose and perpendicular to your face.

2. Extend your lips over your fingers as far as you comfortably can.

3. Inhale deeply and squeeze your fingers tight with the mouth muscle. Squeeze hard and feel the mouth muscle tighten against the fingers.

4. Hold for a count of 6 and exhale.

5. Repeat 10 times

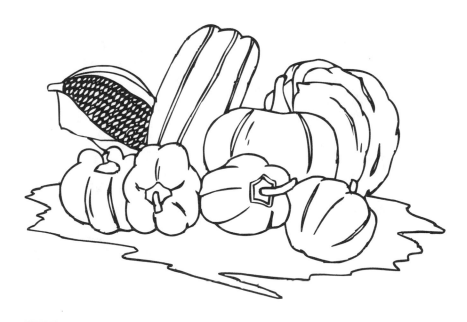

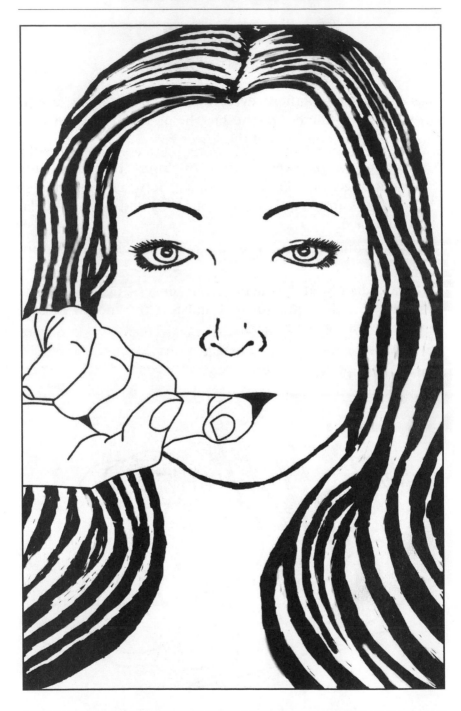

Exercise 10
Squeeze the Knuckle

This exercise tightens the muscles around your mouth and plumps your lips.

1. Wrap the upper lip over the upper teeth and the lower lip over the lower teeth.
2. Place the middle joint of your index finger between your lips. Extend your lips over the knuckle.
3. Take a deep breath and squeeze the knuckle with both lips.
4. Hold for a count of 6.
5. Repeat 10 times.

Try to pull the finger joint out, as if to break free from the grip. This way you will have to hold your grip tighter. That is exactly what will strengthen the *Orbicularis Oris* muscles around your mouth.

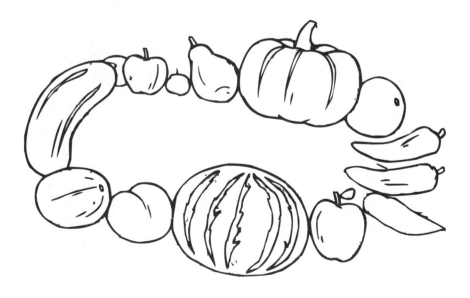

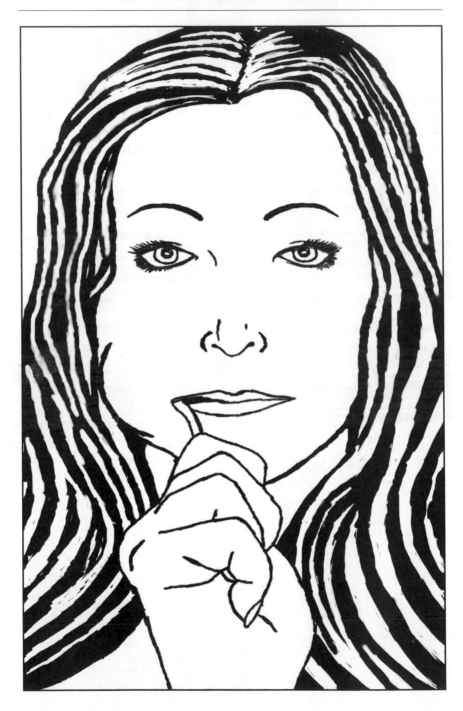

Exercise 11
Cheek Flex

This exercise strengthens the cheek area by building up the *Zygomaticus* muscles.

1. Place a plastic teaspoon inside your mouth with the bowl against the center of your right cheek.
2. Pull the spoon away from your teeth and hold. Your cheek will bulge out like a chipmunk's.
3. Contract the muscles by trying to draw your cheek back to the teeth. Hold to a count of 6.
4. Do the same on the other side.
5. Repeat 10 times.

Using a spoon instead of your finger is not only more convenient, but it seems like a spoon belongs in your mouth and your thumb does not. That's just my preference. Use the thumb of the opposite hand if you like.

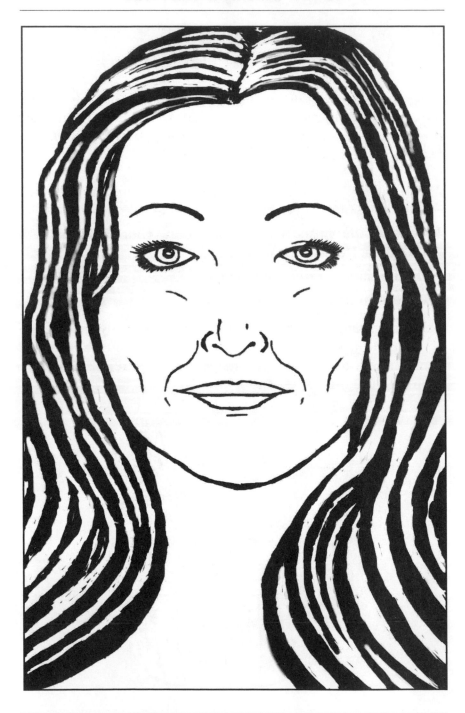

Exercise 12
Smile Push ups for Cheeks

This exercise will re-create the apples of your cheeks, which have a tendency to flatten with age. It will lift the middle portion of your face. It targets the *Quadratus Labii Superioris* muscles.

1. Sit straight and look in a mirror.
2. Using your cheek muscles, pout, (i.e. thrust out your lips) showing as much of your lips as you can.
3. Keeping your lips closed, smile.
4. Suck in your cheeks onto your jaws.
5. Hold this position for a count of 6. You must work these muscles to exhaustion, until you feel they are burning and then relax.
6. Repeat 10 times.

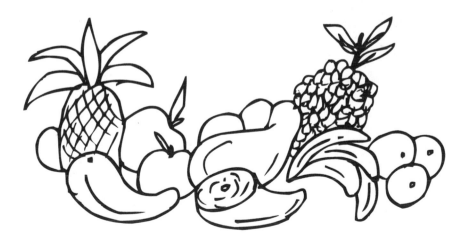

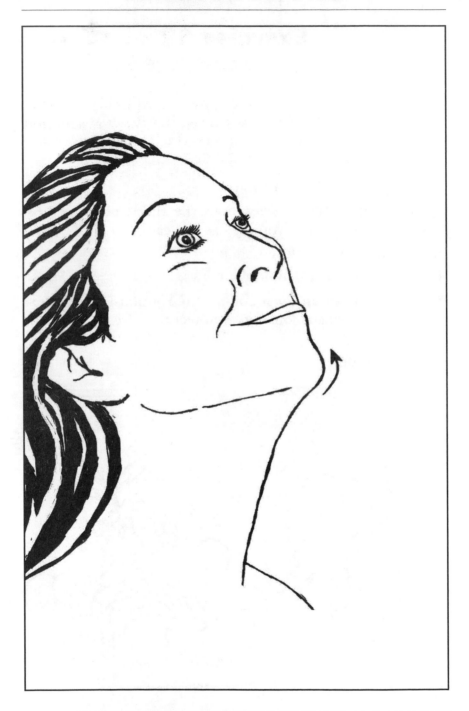

Exercise 13
Grin Exercise

This exercise will develop the bunch of cheek muscles below the eyes. It also strengthens the *Quadratus Labii Superioris* muscles.

1. Pull your bottom lip over your top lip.
2. Tilt your chin slightly upwards until you can feel it pulling on your neck.
3. Open your eyes as wide as possible and grin from ear to ear. You must work these muscles to exhaustion, until you feel they are burning.
4. Hold this position for a count of 6.
5. Repeat 10 times.

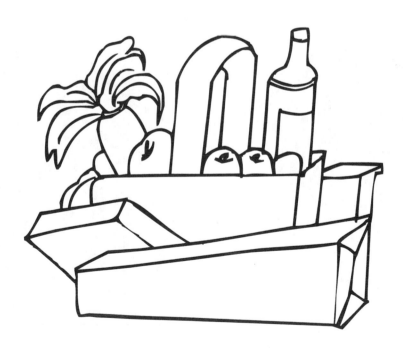

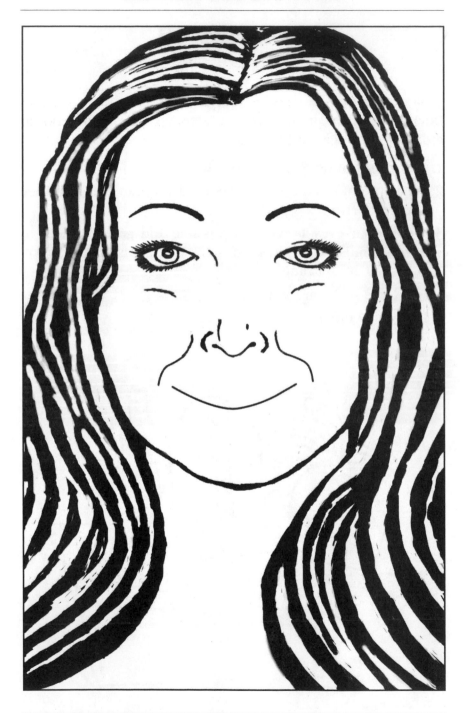

Exercise 14
Tight Smile

This exercise lifts the corners of your mouth. It will diminish jowls (the areas of fullness along the jawline that tend to increase with age) and pouches.

1. Sit straight in front of the mirror.
2. Open your mouth. Wrap the upper lip over the upper teeth and the lower lip over the lower teeth.
3. Press the lips tightly against each other.
4. Now try hard to smile. Hold the smile, no matter how small, for a count of 6. You must work the muscles to exhaustion, until you feel they are burning.
5. Repeat 10 times.

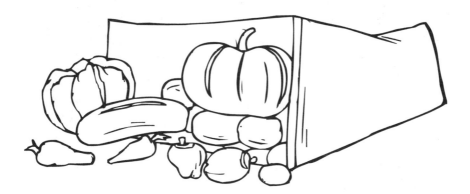

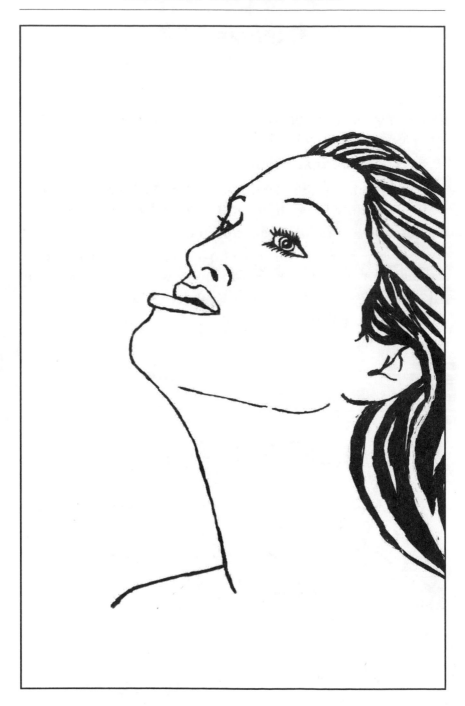

Exercise 15
Scooping Exercise

This exercise targets all muscles of the lower face. It eliminates sagging jowls and pouches. It will decrease a double chin and eventually eliminate it.

1. Lift your head up and tilt your neck back as far as possible. The skin below your chin should be tightening.
2. Open and close your mouth, pulling your lower jaw forward in a scooping motion, as if you are trying to scoop something up with your lower jaw.
3. Hold for a count of 6 in the upper position.
4. Repeat 10 times.

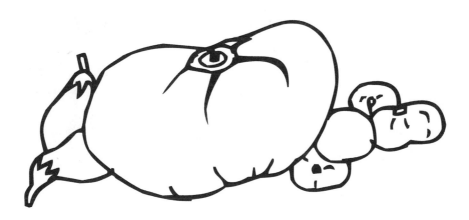

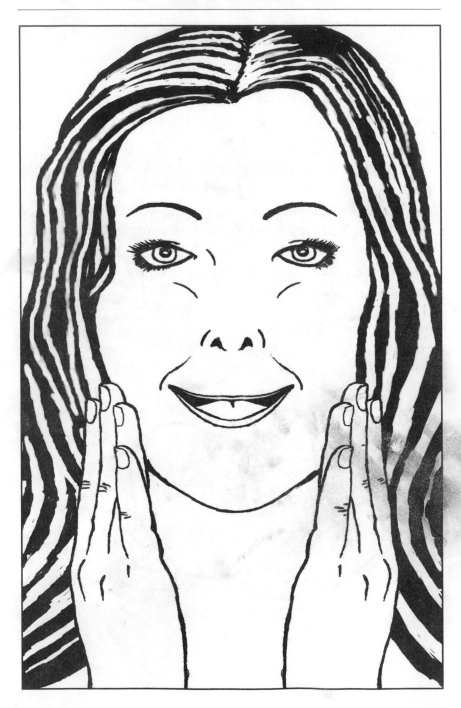

Exercise 16
Slide Your Face

This exercise greatly improves circulation in your face.

1. Sit straight.
2. Open your mouth as wide as comfortable. Wrap the upper lip over the upper teeth and the lower lip over the lower teeth. Smile.
3. Place the three middle fingers of each hand at your jaw line on both sides of your head.
4. Slide your fingers along the sides of your face towards the temples, in a very slow motion at least for a count of 6.
5. Repeat 10 times.

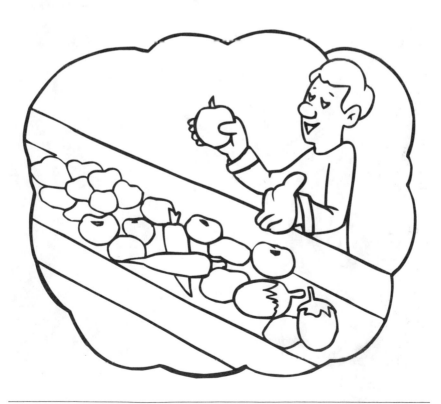

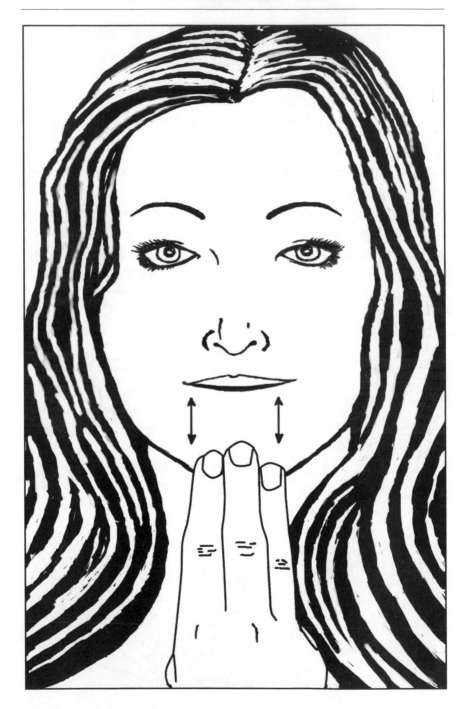

Exercise 17
Chin Lift

This exercise builds up *Mentalis*, the muscles in the chin, giving visual lift and smoothness to the chin area.

1. Sit straight. Tilt your head slightly upward.

2. Take your three middle fingers, place them on the chin vertically and pull the chin down.

3. At the same time, curl the lower lip over the bottom teeth to provide counter resistance.

4. Very slowly repeat motion 10 times.

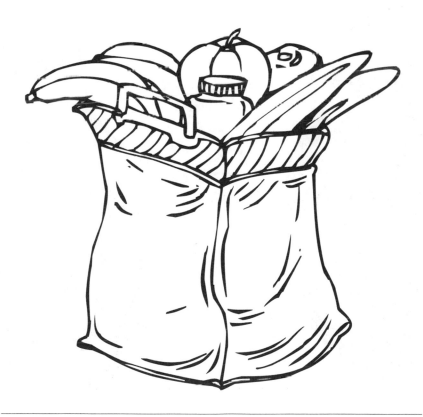

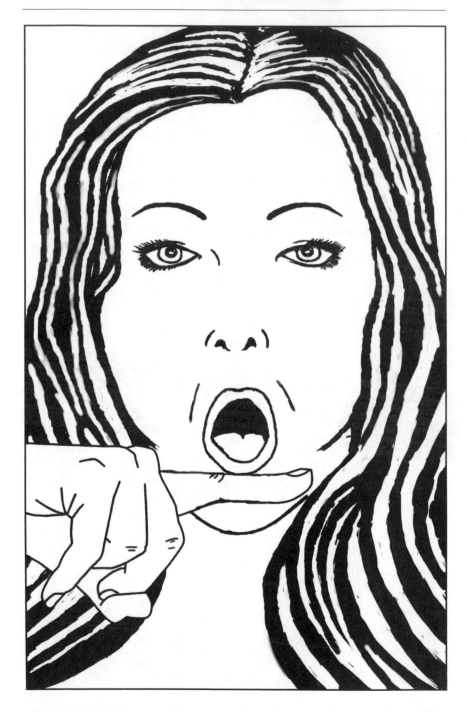

Exercise 18
Jawline Definer

This exercise targets the *Digastricus* muscle, which opens the mouth by depressing the jaw. It will not only firm the under the chin area, but will also prevent bone loss in the lower jaw.

1. Sit straight. Open your mouth as wide as possible.
2. Place the index finger of one hand horizontally on your face below your lips.
3. With the side of your index finger press firmly against your chin. Now try to close your mouth.
4. Very slowly repeat motion 10 times.

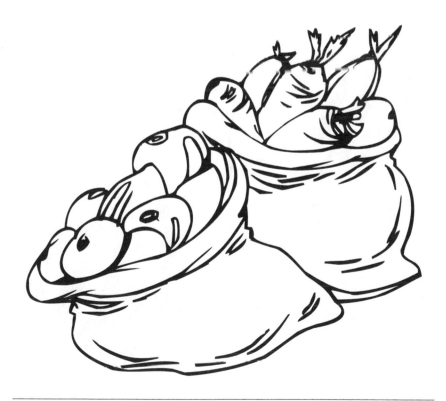

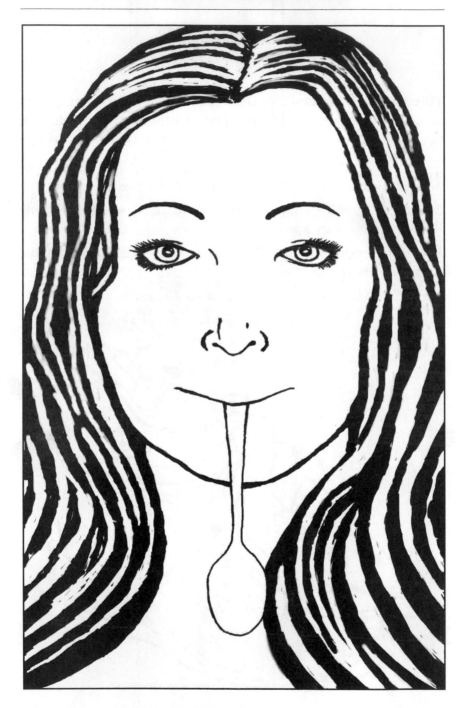

Exercise 19
Upper Jaw Builder

This exercise builds up your upper jaw. It prevents bone loss and can actually reverse the "sunken-mouth" look, a sign of old age.

1. Take a tablespoon. Place the handle part of the spoon into your mouth.
2. Let the other end drop all the way down but still hold it with your facial muscles.
3. Now flex the muscles around your mouth and lift the spoon to the horizontal level.
4. Hold in the horizontal position for a count of 6.
5. Lower the spoon slightly, then raise it again.
6. Repeat 10 times

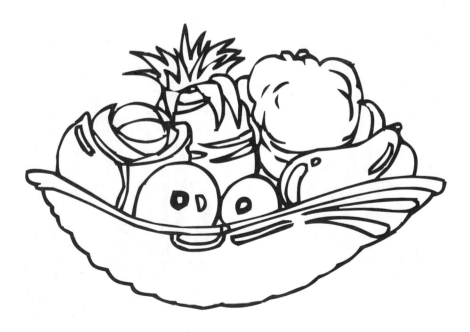

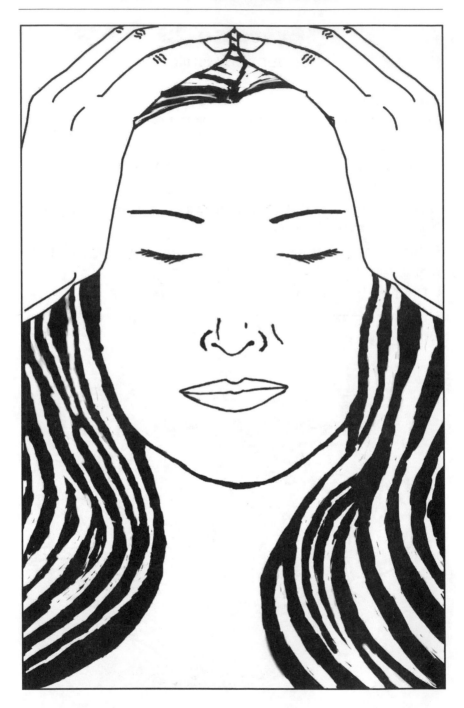

Exercise 20
Crow's Feet

This exercise targets the *Orbicularis Oculi,* the muscles around the eyes. The purpose is to eliminate crow's feet.

1. Lift your eyebrows and place the flat part of your hands beside your eyes, covering the wrinkles, including the edge of the bone. Rest your fingers on the top of your head.
2. Slide the hands from the corners of your eyes towards your temples. Now close your eyes tightly.
3. Hold for a count of 6.
4. Repeat 10 times.

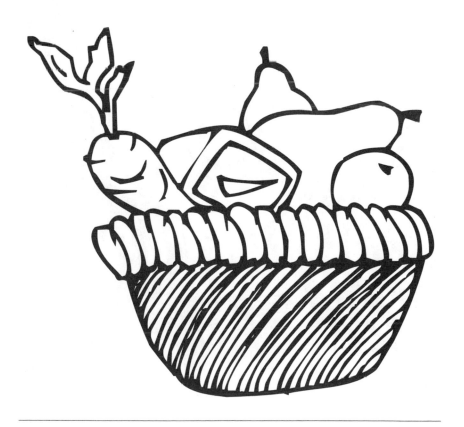

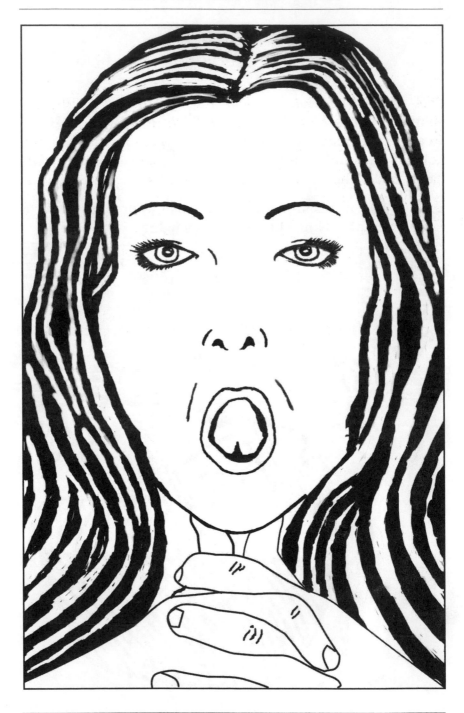

Exercise 21
Tongue Press

This targets the *Mylohyoideus* muscle directly under the chin. The purpose of this exercise is to firm and fill up the area which is most prone to atrophy. This atrophy results in a hollow area under the chin in some people or skin that hangs under the weight of fat in others. This is a simple but crucial exercise to create a more youthful appearance in this area.

1. Sit straight. Lace your fingers together, leaving your thumbs sticking out.

2. Push up on the chin muscle with your thumbs.

3. At the same time, press your tongue to the roof of your mouth. This will cause the chin muscle to push down against your thumbs.

4. Hold it for a count of 6.

5. Repeat 10 times.

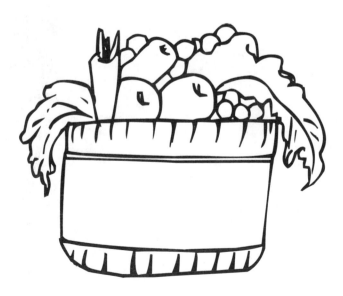

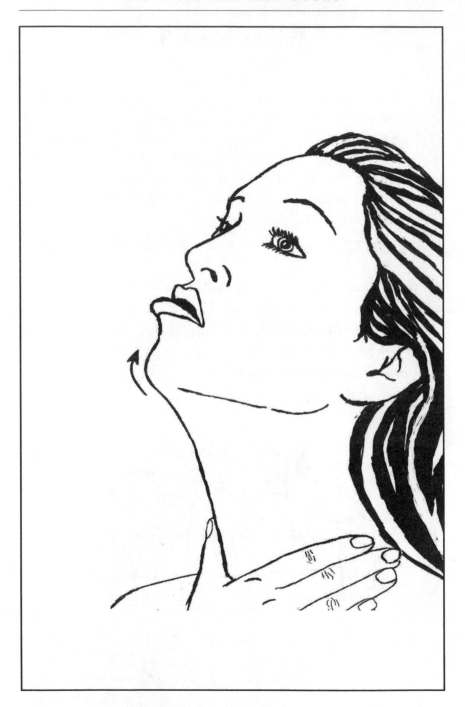

Exercise 22
Fish Mouth Exercise

This exercise is great for firming the chin, neck, and jaw line by strengthening the *Platysma* muscle. The *Platysma* muscle is a large, thin muscle. It is one of the first muscles to wrinkle and droop. This exercise addresses the cords below the neck called "turkey wattles."

1. Sit straight. Place one hand at the base of the throat, over the collarbone, and pull down slightly on the skin with a firm grip.

2. Tilt the head back. Distend the lower lip like a fish gulping for water.

3. Lift the chin up as if you have a load hanging from it.

4. Hold for a count of 6.

5. Repeat 10 times.

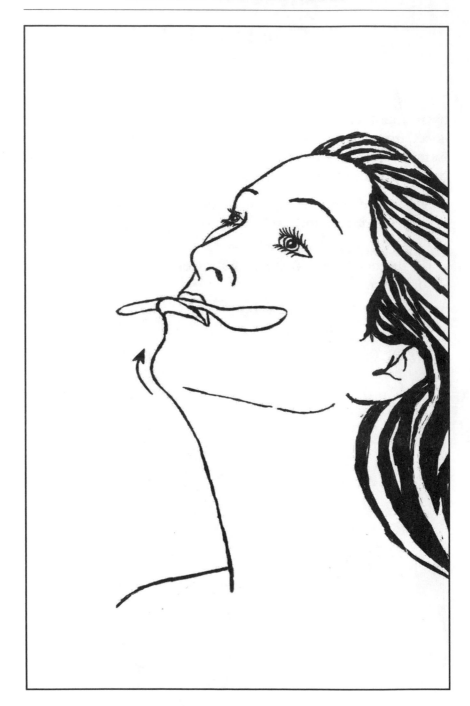

Exercise 23
Chin Push-ups with a Spoon

This is my favorite exercise. It lifts the lower part of your face. You can begin with a teaspoon and then graduate to a tablespoon. At some point, you might be able to use a serving spoon to add extra weight. You will be very proud of yourself when you are able to balance a big spoon.

1. Tilt the head back.
2. Distend the lower lip.
3. Place a spoon across your lip like a dumbbell.
4. Lift the lower lip with the spoon on it up. It will move the chin over your chin bone.
5. Hold in the up position for a count of 6.
6. Repeat 10 times.

Now turn the spoon 180 degrees so that the handle is on the opposite side. Repeat the exercise.

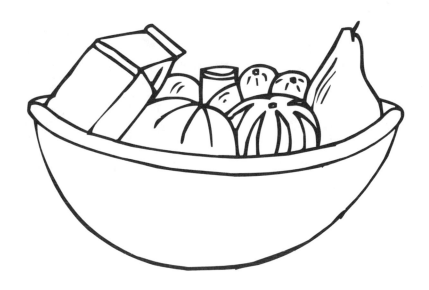

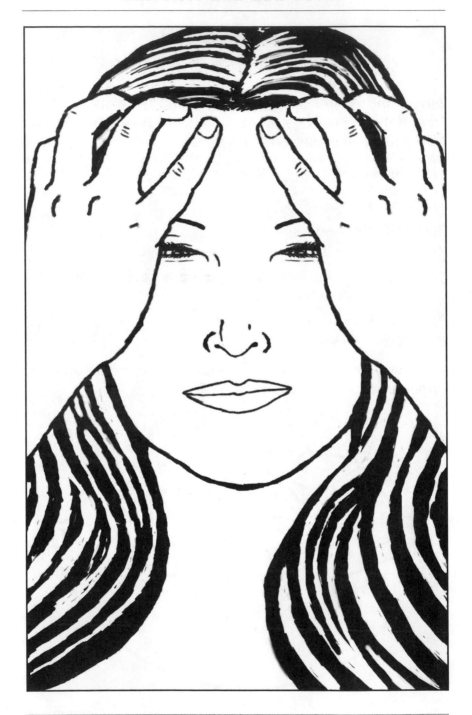

Exercise 24
Brow Smoother

Targets the *Frontalis*, the muscles of the forehead, and the Occipitalis, the muscles in the back of the head. The purpose is to remove lines above the brow.

1. Sit straight. Fan your fingers with your thumbs folded in, and place your fingers where your scalp meets your hair near your temples.
2. Push straight up and press tight.
3. Squint slightly to provide counter resistance.
4. Hold for a count of 6.
5. Repeat 10 times

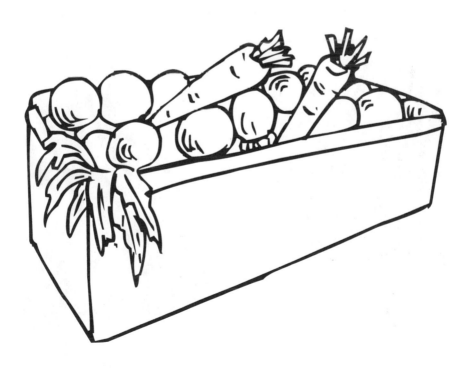

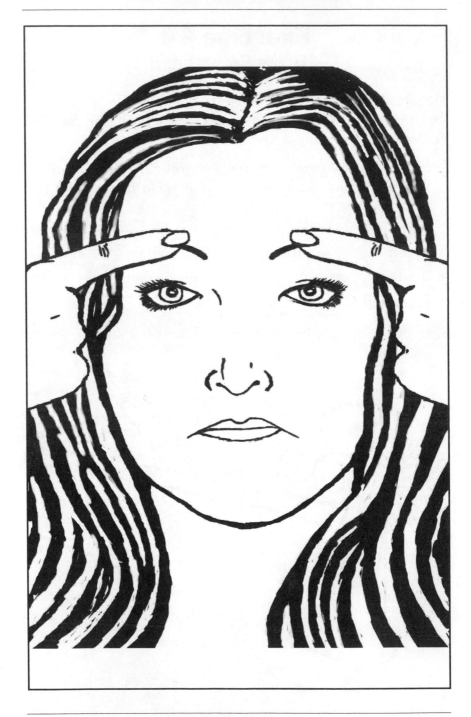

Exercise 25
Frown Furrows Eraser

This two-part exercise targets the *Corrugator Supercilii* and the *Frontalis*, the muscles right above the brow area, to eliminate furrows.

1. Place the tip of each index finger in the center of each eyebrow.
2. Pull the brows apart, and at the same time frown to provide counter resistance.
3. Hold for a count of 6.
4. The second part is just the opposite. Place the tip of each middle finger in the center of each brow and push the brows together (inward).
5. At the same time, raise the eyebrows to provide counter resistance.
6. Hold it for a count of 6.
7. Repeat both parts of the exercise 10 times.

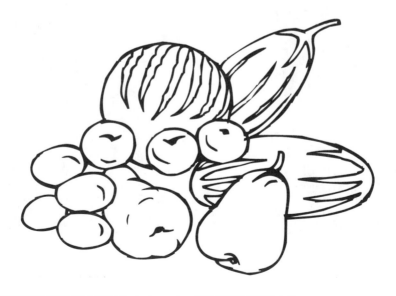

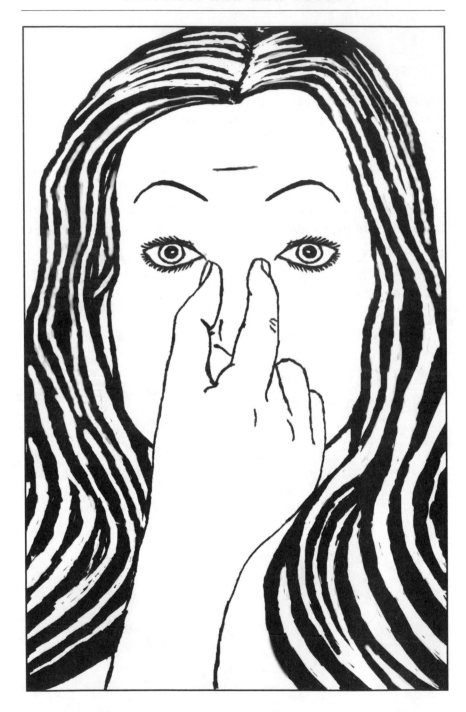

Exercise 26
Bridge of Nose Dewrinkler

This exercise works the *Procerus* muscle and eliminates the wrinkle across the bridge of the nose.

1. With the thumb and the index finger of one hand, hold the skin against the nose bone, across the bridge of the nose, either on the wrinkle you want to eliminate or directly below it.
2. Pull the skin somewhat down and hold this position firmly.
3. Raise your eyebrows to provide counter resistance.
4. Hold it for a count of 6.
5. Repeat 10 times.

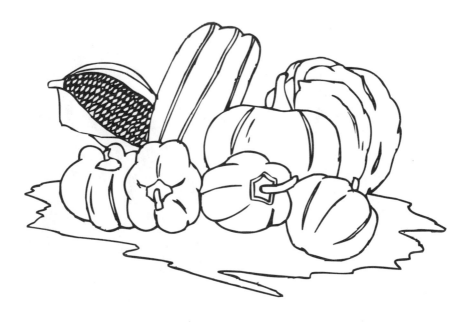

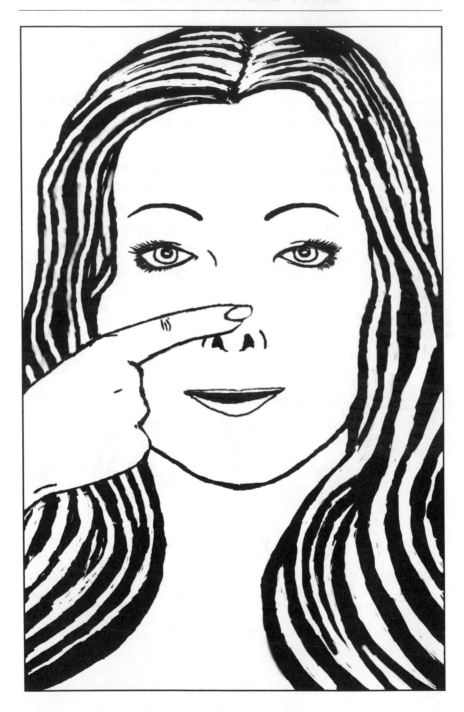

Exercise 27
Nose Shortener

I found this particular exercise in Carole Maggio's book *Facercise*. She was able to correct the dent on her nose, and this technique became one of her signature exercises.

It shortens and narrows the tip of the nose by exercising the *Dilator Naris Posterior* and *Dilator Naris Anterior*, giving your nose a more youthful appearance.

1. Use the index finger to push the tip of the nose up and firmly in place.
2. Flex your nose down by pulling your upper lip down over the teeth.
3. Hold for a count of 6.
4. Repeat 10 times.

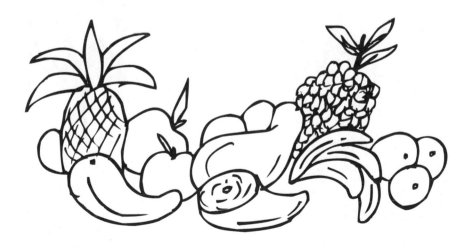

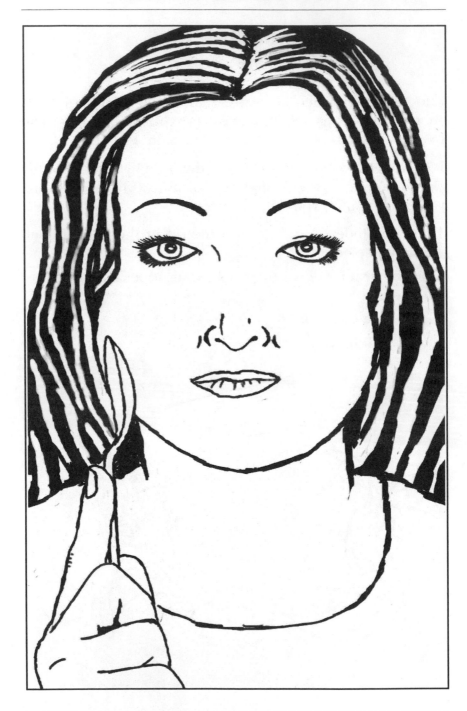

Exercise 28
Cheek Drum

This massaging technique improves elasticity and irons away superficial lines that might have developed with previous exercises.

1. Sit straight facing the mirror.
2. Get as much air in your cheeks as possible. Keep your mouth closed tightly.
3. Now use the back of a spoon to drum gently on both cheeks.
4. For a better effect, place some honey on the back of the spoon and repeat the procedure. The honey is not only very beneficial for your skin, but it will stick to it and will create a little pulling effect as well.

Work your cheeks for at least 30-50 seconds each.

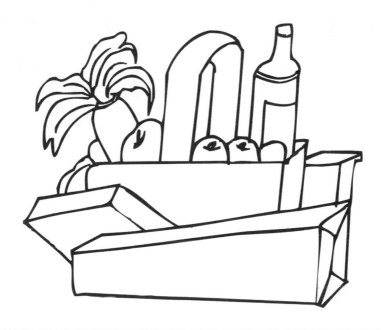

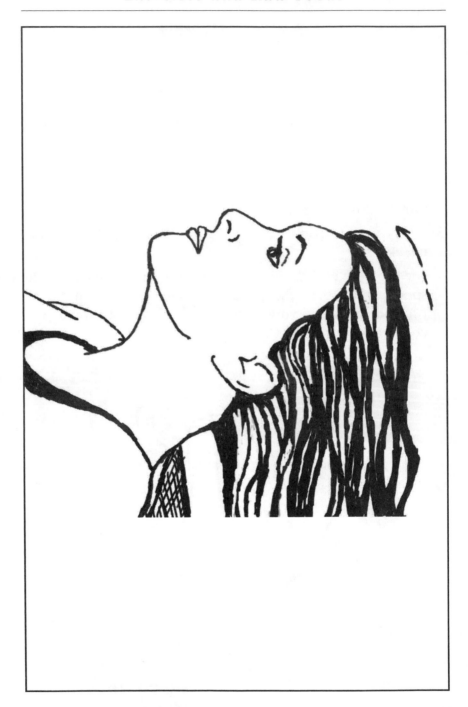

Exercise 29
Neck Smoother

This exercise targets the *Sternocleidomastiodeus,* the major muscle of the neck. When this muscle is increased in size, it elongates the neck, while firming and smoothing the sides of the neck.

1. Lie across a bed, letting your head hang upside down off the side.
2. Raise your head up slowly, stressing the muscles under the jaw.
3. Hold for a count of 6 and lower your head.
4. Repeat 3–5 times.

This is an extremely important exercise for your neck, because that is where aging will show first. But be careful not to overdo it the first several days or you will end up with a sore, stiff neck and shoulders. You must learn to relax your shoulders during this exercise. This will only come with regular practice.

Eventually your goal will be 20–30 repetitions, but do what you can. The exercise will strengthen the neck and lessen the appearance of neck lines. It will also reduce double chins, since they are partially the result of slack neck muscles.

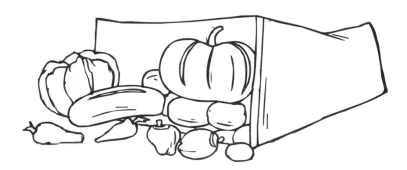

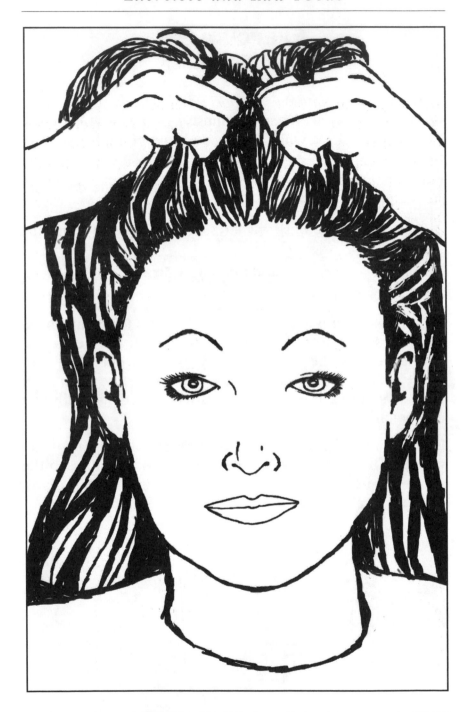

Exercise 30
Face Lift

Grab a big handful of hair and pull gently upwards. It is an extremely good exercise to rejuvenate your face. Even though there is no weight bearing effect, it is literally yoga for your face. Grasp the hair with your fingers, pulling gently, and changing the position of your hands until every part of the scalp has been treated. During this hair pulling process, the skin of the scalp is slightly raised from the skull. Its minute muscles and capillaries are stimulated. This exercise has a general tonic effect, as it stimulates circulation. Applied for short periods of time, stress sends nutrients to the roots of your hair and improves their growth.

Apply *Your Right to Be Beautiful Cream* now. Be sure to use the cream around your eyes to avoid creases.

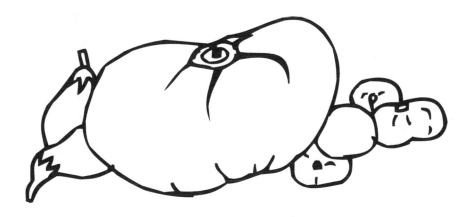

Do Not Have Time To Do Facial Exercises? I Have a Solution!

There are days when I think I am the busiest person in the whole world, although I am sure some of you can challenge me. My day already feels like 25 hours, so I had a serious dilemma regarding how I could find another 20 minutes to work in facial exercises. Where there is a problem, there is a solution. I came up with an idea for simplifying my raw food preparation. (And no, living on air was not an option, plus it wouldn't be original: others have already suggested it.)

I believe that some people who will be attracted to my *Rawsome Flex* book may not have much experience with raw foods. Still, I find it very hard to write for beginners, because I said everything I know about raw foods in my other books, and I definitely don't want to repeat myself.

I found a simple trick to free up 20 minutes, and I am going to share it with you, with the condition that you will use the extra time to do facial exercises. The method is quite simple and will be very useful for beginners, but it may only be appreciated by the raw food veterans, who will recognize a good preparation technique when they see it.

I stumbled on this method through sheer desperation and the severe pressure of not having enough hours in a day. I make 12 ounces of my morning juice and drink only 8 ounces, leaving 4 ounces and making a soup by chopping some vegetables for the second meal. This way my all-raw food preparation takes no more time than making a glass of juice and cutting up a few greens and veggies.

Throughout this book, I present some very easy and delicious soups that you can make with the unused portions of your morning juice. And you old timers thought there was no new way to skin a cat. Now you cannot complain that you have no time to do the exercises. In the following days you will see several recipes to get you started, but I encourage you to improvise and come up with your own as well.

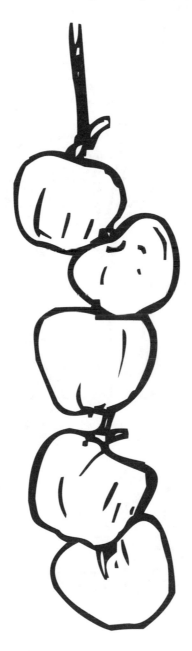

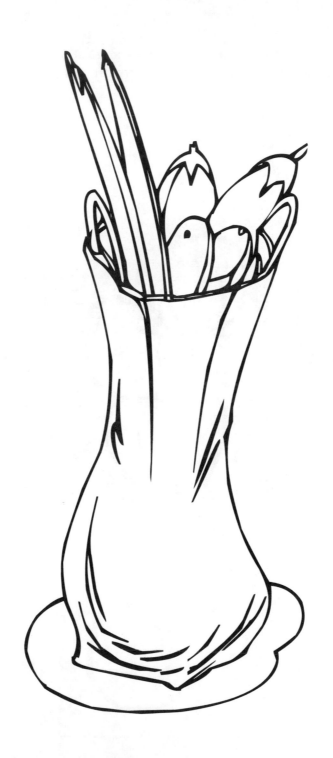

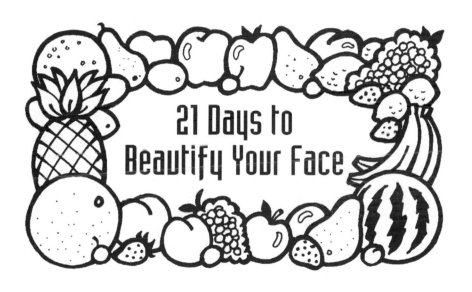

21 Days to Beautify Your Face

To attain the best results, make an effort to read the remainder of the book on a day-by-day basis and follow the instructions as specified. Different exercises will be added on various days to where by day 21 you will be doing all the exercises. Utilizing the 21 day facial exercise initiation program will keep you from becoming overwhelmed and help you to develop a new habit for life.

Day 1

Wrinkles are the result of facial muscles stretching and going soft. The underlying structure no longer supports the skin—gravity at its finest! General wear and tear, and bad facial habits when it comes to daily expressions, emphasize the wrinkles which are inclined to come along with all the sags and bags of age-driven gravity. After thousands and thousands of squints and smiles, the muscles lack sufficient elasticity and strength to return to their former short length. The face falls, along with everything else. Those muscles can stretch half an inch or more by age 55. How scary is that?

Your facial muscles go soft, losing their firmness because the muscles have weakened and can no longer maintain resilience. Skin care regimens keep the skin well maintained, but no cream effectively counters wrinkles. Exercise does. Because cells are renewed with healthy new cells, firming facial exercises can make these fibers grow stronger.

Yoga, it's now widely acknowledged, is excellent for exercising the internal, involuntary muscles. Yoga postures place organs in different anatomical positions, squeezing and stretching them within certain limitations. Organs are supplied with fresh blood, gently massaged, relaxed, and toned into a state of optimum health. Why should facial muscles, even though mostly voluntary, be any different? From this day forward do exercise 30 twice a day.

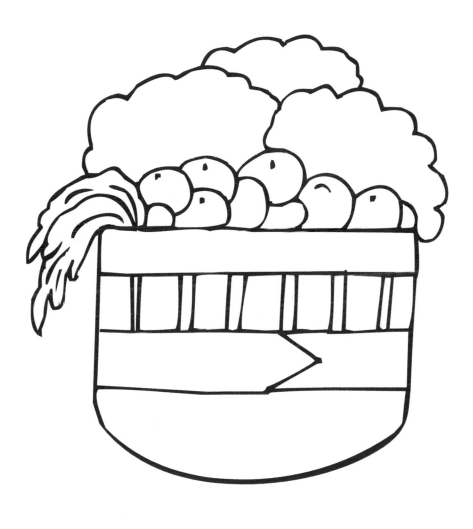

Day 2

What happens to your face when you perform facial exercises? Muscles are strengthened and skin is revitalized by blood flow. Your whole face becomes refreshed. The early starter benefits the most by delaying initial atrophy. But the most obvious results are in men and women 45 and up. Sun damage and advanced aging caused by protein-heavy diets do present serious problems, but even these individuals will see improvements. Those on raw food see even better results because their systems are able to flush out toxins and improve oxygen flow and nutrient distribution to the skin.

The *Rolling Bed of Pins,* available at www.beautifulonraw.com, is a valuable aid in increasing circulation as well. You can use it before or after your exercises.

Like all exercises, facial workouts have to be done regularly. In the beginning, it is recommended that you perform these exercises consecutively for 6 days, with one day given over to "R and R"—you'll need a day of rest just as much as those big Russian weightlifters do! Don't let the experts scare you away. Any exercise is good, and you will be better looking than if you never tried it at all. Continue doing exercise 30 twice a day.

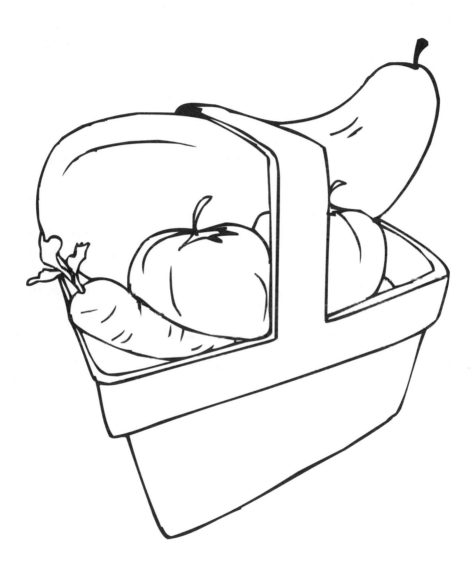

Day 3

You may see some improvement in as little as a week, depending on your state of health and initial damage. After three weeks, most people will feel a difference to the touch. The face shows more tautness and the cheeks become fuller, with more definition in the lips. But let's be realistic...as with all exercise programs, facial progress is basically a slow procedure. Improvements will definitely be noted within 6 weeks but you may need up to a year to achieve optimum results. On the plus side, consider how easy this regimen is— no baggy pants, no sweat, and no pricey gym membership! Once you get where you'd like to be, you'll find that maintenance requires at least three days a week for as long as you want to keep your new, improved face.

In the meantime, begin consuming cucumbers whenever possible to nourish your skin from the inside. Read my book *Beautiful on Raw: Uncooked Creations* for more information on the beauty enhancing qualities of raw foods. Include one of these recipes in your menu as desired:

From *Beautiful on Raw: Uncooked Creations*:

Complexion Clarifier

4 pickle-size cucumbers

3 stalks celery

2 medium carrots

2 medium apples

2 handfuls fresh spinach

Juice all ingredients and drink immediately.

OR

Emerald Skin Silk

1 mango, peeled and pitted

1 banana

½ medium cucumber

¼ pineapple, cored and peeled

Place all ingredients in a blender with 1 cup water and blend until smooth.

Continue doing exercise 30 twice a day. From this day forward do exercise 1 twice a day as well.

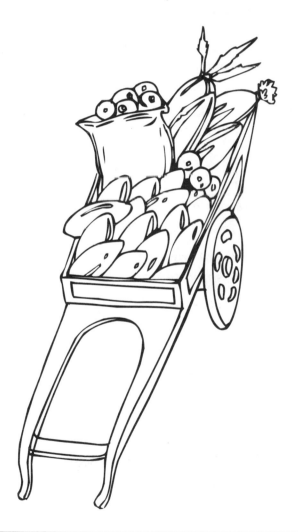

Day 4

Facial muscles are unlike most other muscles in the body. Muscles in your legs and arms are attached to bone at both ends. One end of a facial muscle, however, attaches to skin or to another muscle. Resistance contractions help tighten and lift the contours of the face, giving a more youthful look.

Six areas require concentrated exercises to improve their appearance: forehead, eyes, cheeks, lips, neck, and chin. These areas overlap, of course, but we will consider them separately as essential areas as the program unfolds.

Make this Green Smoothie recipe from Victoria Boutenko's book *Green for Life*, available on www.beautifulonraw.com.

> ### Green Benevolence
>
> *6-8 leaves of Romaine lettuce*
>
> *1 cup of red grapes*
>
> *1 orange*
>
> *1 banana*
>
> *2 cups water*
>
> *Place all ingredients in a blender and blend until smooth. Makes about 1 quart.*

Continue doing exercises 1 and 30 twice a day.

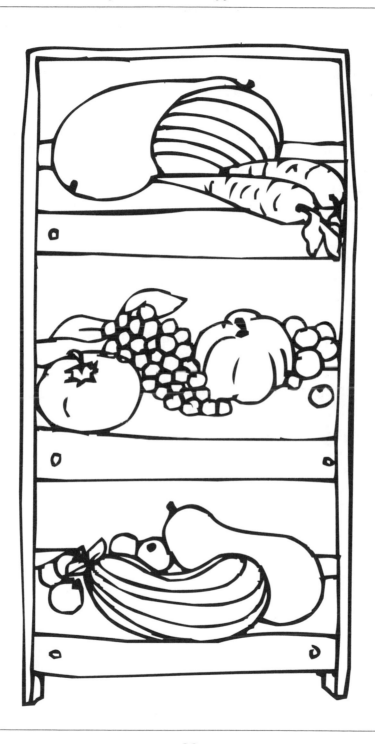

Day 5

Forehead...Your forehead runs from your hairline to your eyebrows. You can think of the forehead in vertical terms even though we are inclined to think it is horizontal, since that is definitely the way it falls. Atrophy, along with gravity, stretches the muscle and lets the eyebrows gradually droop over the eyes, deepening horizontal creases in this once-smooth area. These are facial muscles that do not respond so much to lack of activity as to emotional expressions. The more animated your emotional expressions, the more likely you are to have "expression lines."

Beauty queens, models, TV personalities, and others who depend on their faces are regularly trained not to move their facial muscles so they will not create lines or wrinkles. Think about actresses. "Character actresses" are those who have interesting faces. Stars are the ones who look permanently Botoxed (whether they are or not). There should be a happy medium.

Read my book *Your Right to Be Beautiful* for information about avoiding expression lines.

From this day forward, you will do exercises 24 and 25 twice a day (along with exercise 1 and 30).

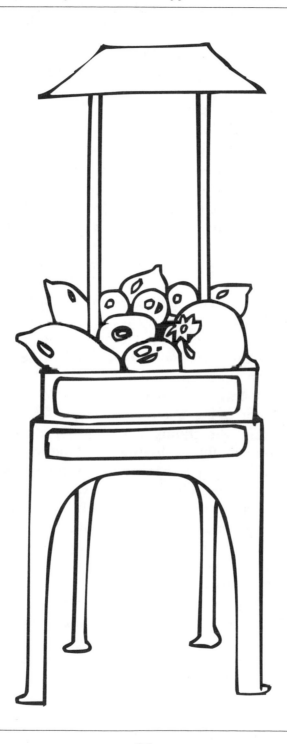

Day 6

Eyes...Your eyes are affected by the downward slide of your eyebrows. They slide off the brow bone and cause the upper eye to become heavier—the so-called "hooded eye." Others can't see your eyes, and sometimes you can't see out. Let this continue on its downward slide, and eventually your vision will be impaired. Drooping eyes make you look tired, angry, worn out. Your eyebrows fall over the dark eye shadow the cosmetic companies tell you to put in the crease below your brow to bring out your eyes. All this collapse makes the eyes appear smaller instead.

Then there are the dreaded crow's feet, caused by squinting—something we all do in the sun or when reading fine print, or just when smiling. Exercising the essential eye muscles can eliminate most of these lines.

The eyes have been called the "windows of the soul." They are also the window to youth. Since the eyes are so essential to emotion and interaction, any deterioration in their elasticity relays a negative message of tiredness and depression. Your upper eyelids are subject to two different forms of aging, depending on your facial musculature. Atrophy causes the lids to disappear behind the eyeballs. The more familiar and probably more unattractive look is caused by stretching, sagging skin that blurs eye definition.

The area under the eye is also subject to two different aging processes. One leads to that hollow-eyed appearance caused by the loss of the flesh padding under the eye. The other, more noticeable if not more prevalent, is the infamous "luggage" look. Bags are caused by fluid collecting under the eye because of poor circulation. This, too, can be corrected with exercise. When the fat pads in the eye socket weaken, fat drifts forward, filling the sensitive area under eyes.

From this day forward, add exercises 2 through 5 to your twice a day facial exercise routine.

Try this juice recipe from *Beautiful on Raw: Uncooked Creations:*

Eyebag Remover

1 small beet (beet root and beet greens)

3 celery stalks

2 medium apples

½ small organic lemon with the skin still on (you should cut the lemon in half first to remove the seeds)

Juice all ingredients and drink immediately.

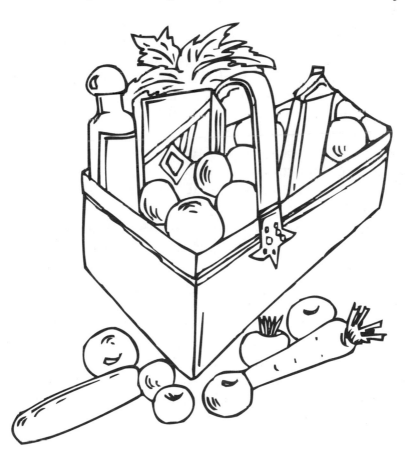

Day 7

My "Cheek Flex" was inspired by Deborah Crowley. After watching her DVD, I found that it was her cheek exercises I remembered most vividly. First, they proved effective. Second, she used her thumbs, placing them into her mouth to create the designated effect. I used to think: What a pity I won't be able to do them. I wear my nails long. I'm proud of my nails. Nails tell a story about your health. I practically never break a nail. I have to cut them when they get too long. I knew I would not want to wear them short even to benefit my face. I had to find another way. And I did.

The solution was very simple…an ordinary spoon. Once I began thinking about spoons of different sizes, other amazing possibilities emerged. I was so proud that I discovered how to use spoons in my facial exercise program that I wanted to see how original my idea was. Not entirely, as it turns out. There really is nothing entirely new under the sun.

I learned that German cosmetologist Renee Cox developed a special massage done with spoons. But I've innovated. Let me present to you the most effective techniques I've found. I've chosen the best from the best, adding my own insights and revelations acquired through painstaking investigation.

From this day forward add exercise 11 to your twice a day facial exercise routine.

Try the following recipe:

Blended Curry in a Hurry

In the morning juice:

2-4 carrots

4 stalks celery

1 apple

a 1-inch piece of ginger root

Refrigerate approximately 1 cup and drink the remaining juice.

For your lunch, combine in blender:

1 cup of the leftover juice

1 avocado

1 Tablespoon of curry powder

Pour into a bowl and garnish with a handful of chopped fresh cilantro or spinach.

Celtic salt to taste

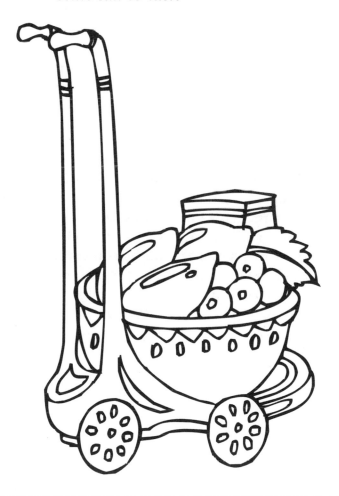

Day 8

The loss of muscle tone is not the only cause of wrinkles and sagging skin. Many other factors contribute to the sagging and drooping of the skin: deteriorating collagen and elastin, depletion of the skin's fat layer, sagging muscle due to the loosening of facial ligaments holding the muscles in place, hormonal changes, depleted collagen production, thinning of the skin due to free radical damage, genetic disposition, and poor diet can all produce sagging, discolored, dull skin.

These are problems that raw foods can help solve. Raw foods restore the worn-out collagen, elastin, and the skin's fat layer. If someone tells you this is impossible, it is because they have never done raw foods. How would they know?

Face exercise experts like Santa Maria Runge, Deborah Crowley, Carole Maggio, and Carolyn Cleaves have developed very good exercise programs. Santa Maria Runge developed her program in her late twenties, Deborah Crowley and Carole Maggio in their thirties. Carolyn Cleaves improved her face appearance in her late fifties *without* the benefit of a raw food regimen. On the raw foods lifestyle, I never even needed such a program until I was 50. I thought: "If these other women could take ten years off their faces *without* raw foods, how much more could be achieved by combining a raw foods regimen *and* facial exercises?" The results, I knew, may prove amazing.

For step-by-step guidance on how to make the transition to a raw foods diet, read my e-book *100 Days to 100% Raw.*

From this day forward, add exercise 21 to your twice a day facial exercise routine.

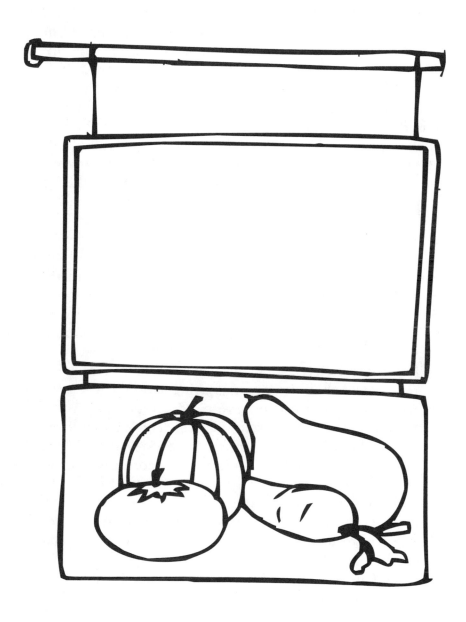

Day 9

Cheeks…Like the eyes, your cheeks have two areas that can age and must be treated differently. The upper cheek muscles are secured to the hairline, while the group of twelve muscles at the other end comes together under the mouth muscles. These are fairly heavy muscles, by facial standards, and when gravity wins, you get jowls, a down-turned mouth, and deep creases from nose to chin. The end effect of all this downward travel can also follow the lower cheeks, adding what appears to be pounds of flesh to the lower half of the face. This process accounts for about 50% of the aging appearance. The good news is, these muscles respond very well to exercises by giving an impression of high cheek bones and lifting the whole face. Another very broad and strong muscle underlies these cheek-supporting muscles. It, too, is fastened along the jawbone. This may be termed the chewing muscle, and, while it plays an important part in supporting the cheeks and determining their contour, it cannot be contracted or exercised at will, except in the act of chewing.

Do all the exercises. But now, when doing exercises 12, 13 and 14, you should add a massaging action. These are voluntary muscles and can be exercised "voluntarily." You can contract these cheek muscles at will. This action forms a clump on the cheekbones under the eyes. While the cheek muscles are contracted, they should be vigorously massaged. Here's how to do it. Press firmly with the palm of the hand on your cheek and rub these bunched muscles firmly and deliberately towards the temples. I sometimes like to use my knuckles instead of my palms. After massaging one cheek, repeat on the other. Or if you prefer, do both at once. This exercise delivers good results in quick time. But persistence and daily workouts are musts.

From this day forward add exercises 12 through 14 to your twice a day facial exercise routine.

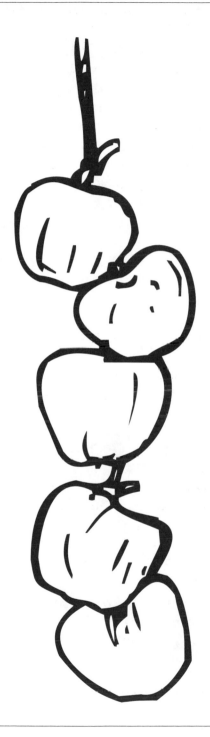

Day 10

Lips…While everything above is heading below, the lips get caught in the avalanche and practically disappear. Unlike other muscles, the lips do not elongate, but shrivel up through lack of circulation. As with everything that shrivels, lips become thinner and wrinkles appear, causing lipstick to wander into uncharted territory.

To reverse this situation, start adding exercises 7 through 10 to your twice a day routine.

Tasty Taco Soup

In the morning juice:

4-5 ripe tomatoes

2 stalks celery

1 carrot

1 peeled lemon

Refrigerate approximately 1 cup and drink the remaining juice.

For your lunch:

Pour leftover juice into a bowl and top with the following:

small handful of fresh (not boiled!) corn kernels (slice them right off the cob)

chopped tomato

chopped red pepper

¼ onion

dusting of taco seasoning or chili powder (optional)

oregano

Dash of Celtic sea salt

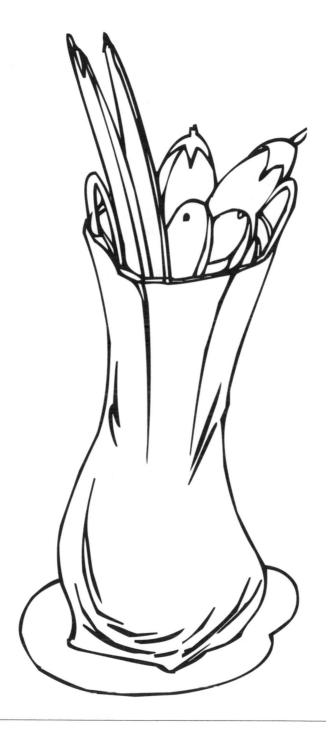

Day 11

Neck...The neck, which goes from the lower cheek to the upper chest, is the largest muscle involved in facial aging. When the neck muscle ages, the result can be a "turkey wattle"—a loose flap of skin hanging beneath the chin. This is not to be confused with the pouchy area directly under the jawline—the so-called double chin. There are actually two different types of double chins. One is caused by fatty deposits which result from obesity and can be eliminated *only* by improving your diet and thereby losing weight. The double chin caused by tired, sagging muscles *can* be helped by exercise.

From this day forward, add exercises 6, 22 and 23 to your twice a day routine.

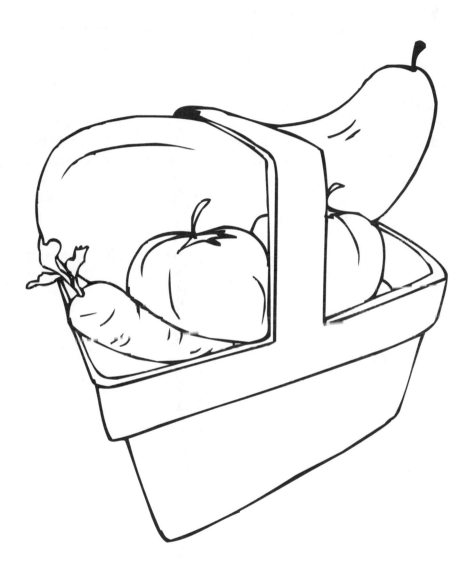

Day 12

Be sure to use Multi-Herbal Green Clay Masque every morning. I apply it first thing upon awakening.

Here is a beauty tip to make the most of the time you keep your masque on: After you have applied the masque: Lie on your back with your knees bent so the small of your back is in contact with the mattress at all times. Hang your head slightly over edge of the bed. At first, start with your head and neck flat on the bed, then inch your body toward the edge of the bed just until your neck begins to bend. Make sure the edge of your bed supports the nape of your neck. It is very important to breathe deeply. Remain in this position for 4-5 minutes. While the masque is working on your face this position allows your facial muscles to counteract gravity and for new blood to rush to your face.

This is the best time to do exercise 29. Add it to your twice a day routine.

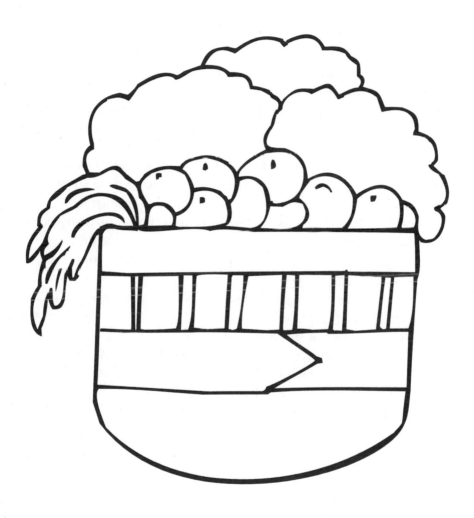

Day 13

Chin and Jaw...If no pressure is applied to the bone it will be re-absorbed so that precious calcium can be deposited elsewhere. The jawbone begins to dissolve, resulting in concave surfaces, causing that sunken-mouth look. This sunken appearance to the lower face makes us look older than we actually are. Bone loss also contributes to deep wrinkling, a pointed chin and jowls, and reduction in biting strength. It could be concluded that the lack of hard chewing because of missing teeth, crowns, or other dental work adversely affects the growth and development of the jaw.

Only the jawbone that has chewed often and hard retains its form. Here is another reason to eat your salad: Chewing your raw greens, vegetables, and roots is good for your beauty! The exercises will help prevent bone atrophy and shrinking gums. These simple exercises will bring fullness to drooping, wrinkled, and sagging lips and help to restore normal facial aesthetics.

The muscles that cover and round the chin are, in most cases, involuntary. That is to say, without practice these muscles are incapable of motion at will. The chin muscles may be classed as involuntary and can be developed only by massage. Broad, flat, muscular bands start under the jawbone and run upward towards the cheekbones, covering the jaws to which they are attached. If these coverings shrink, as they usually do with age, the skin hangs loose. To offset this effect, the massaging technique described below should be practiced along the edge of the jawbone using the heel of your hand. Deep, firm rubbing of the jaw muscles will develop these muscles.

Massage procedure: Rest your chin on the palms of your hands, press up firmly with your hands, and rub the underlying muscles vigorously. For rapid muscle growth, be sure to shift the position of the hands. The continuous pressure must be alternated with short periods of relaxation. This treatment will speedily tone these muscles and increase their size, thus giving a rounder and more youthful appearance to the lines of the jaws.

From this day forward add exercises 17, 18 and 19 to your twice a day routine.

Check out *Belt of Pins*. It can be worn around your head under your chin. Using your *Belt of Pins* will increase blood flow and lymph drainage in applied areas, aiding the removal of fluids and toxins. When you target specific areas of your body, the pins increase the breakdown of fat and cellulite while speeding up fat metabolism. When worn regularly, the

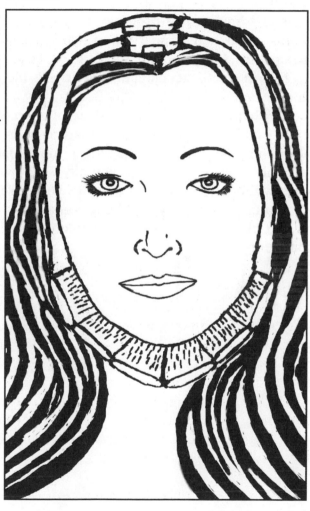

pins will liquefy fat and then slowly release it into the capillaries and lymphatic system.

Day 14

Facial exercises improve circulation, drawing bacteria and toxins to your skin's surface for easier removal. Some people might notice minor spots or blemishes appearing after starting facial exercises. Don't panic. This is quite normal and should be welcomed as a part of the detox process. Your skin is stimulated to produce its natural oils and lubricants. Minor spots may appear when starting facial exercises until toxins are removed and the skin is functioning efficiently. Cell turnover is accelerated and these blemishes will soon disappear.

With proper exercises and a sound raw foods regimen, new cells are produced and mature cells are activated to function with renewed vigor. After you do facial exercises for a while, you will begin to actually *feel* your facial muscles. You will become aware of muscles you never knew you had.

Your slimmed face will be a bonus.

From this day forward add exercise 15 to your twice a day routine.

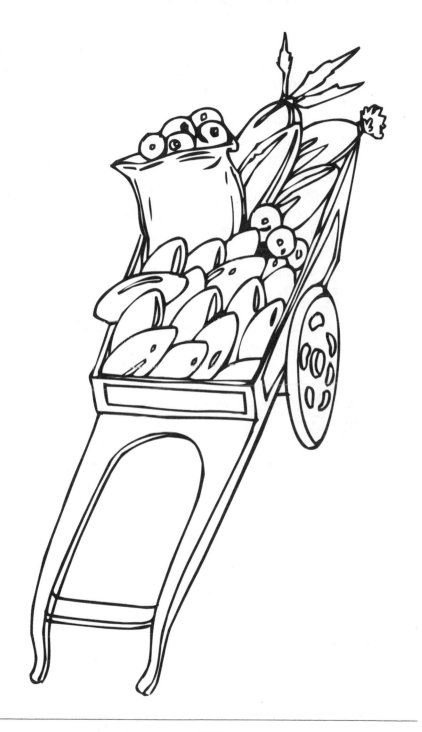

Day 15

Spoon Massage…Put a spoon in crushed ice. This chilling will help your skin's elasticity, eliminate eye bags, and make any dark circles under your eyes less visible. Another useful long-term effect is the strengthening of your vision through stimulation of the area around your eyes.

Spoons can be applied to the base of the eyebrows, where a circular motion near the temples helps smooth wrinkles on the forehead, relieving tension and stimulating the brain. To make the skin more elastic at the neck, use your spoon in a rotating motion from the chin to the base of the neck. In the course of a spoon massage, acupressure points are activated. One tip: You should apply an ice-cold spoon to the eye area only if you do not have any irritation in that area.

Want to iron out those wrinkles? Use a spoon warmed in a hot water. Be careful not to burn yourself. Test on the back of your hand first. Apply cream to your skin before you apply your spoon.

From this day forward add exercise 28 to your twice a day routine.

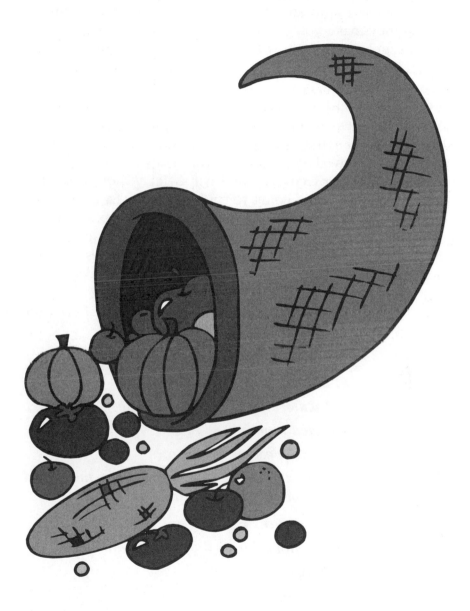

Day 16

The most important by-product of doing facial exercises is that they make you develop a renewed awareness of your face. Regular exercise will eventually help your muscles relax. This might at first seem counterproductive, since the point of exercise is a tightening and toning process that gives your muscles better shape. But facial exercises have two parts—flexing and relaxing. Through relaxation, angry expression lines and crow's feet begin to soften, and future lines will be staved off.

Watching your face over time will quickly show you what expressions are really going to "ugly up" your face and how you got those lines in the first place—for example, by squinting or frowning. Facial exercise will hone your muscle awareness and you'll be able to relax those muscles *without* being pumped full of some ghastly paralytic drug (i.e. Botox).

From this day forward add exercises 26 and 27 to your twice a day routine.

> ### *Refreshing Fruit Bowl*
>
> *In the morning juice:*
>
> *1/2 watermelon (or 1 small one)*
>
> *1 peeled lime*
>
> *a 1-inch piece of ginger root*
>
> *Refrigerate approximately 1 cup or more and drink the remaining juice.*
>
> *For your lunch:*
>
> *Pour leftover juice into a bowl and add:*
>
> *1 chopped mango*
>
> *1 sliced banana*
>
> *fresh blueberries or raspberries (optional)*

fresh chopped mint
a drizzle of raw honey, if desired

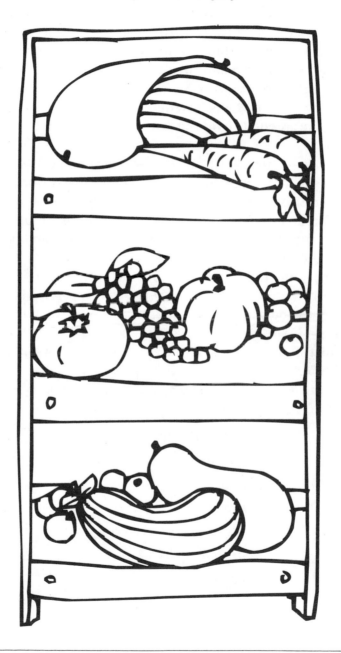

Day 17

Do not ignore the power of your mind to help your progress. For example, a study discussed in the November 24, 2001 issue of *New Scientist* magazine found that when researchers asked volunteers to imagine flexing one of their biceps as hard as possible five times a week, the volunteers who thought about exercise showed a 13.5% increase in strength after a few weeks. The control group who missed out on the mental workout showed no improvement in strength.

Visualize your cheek muscles strengthening. *See* in your mind's eye that "runway model, high cheekbones effect" developing. *Feel* muscles growing, making your skin smooth and firm. Imagine wrinkles and facial lines disappearing. Imagine improved circulation of your blood, giving you a radiant complexion.

There's nothing magic, nothing "unscientific" here. Motivation matters in any long-term effort. Keep visualizing. Keep exercising. As they say in addiction recovery programs, "it works—if you work it."

From this day forward add exercise 20 to your twice a day routine.

You can find more information about intention and visualization in my latest book *Quantum Eating*.

Zesty Skin Food

In the morning juice:

3 parsnips

4 carrots

1 red pepper

1 cucumber

2 stalks celery

1 peeled lemon

Refrigerate approximately 1 cup and drink the remaining juice.

For your lunch:

Put leftover juice into a bowl and garnish with one or all:

chopped tomatoes

chopped spinach

shredded romaine lettuce

a small handful of soaked pistachios

dash of Celtic sea salt

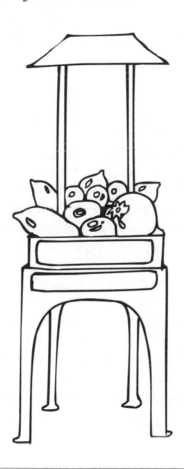

Day 18

Recently I came across an old book written by Sanford Bennett—*Old Age Its Cause and Prevention: The Story of an Old Body and Face Made Young.* In his book, Bennett presents pictures of himself at fifty and at seventy-two. The transformation was remarkable—and we're talking way before Photoshop.

Most of Bennett's book is devoted to exercises done in bed. These are exceptionally good. I wish I had known about them when I was recovering from my hip replacement surgeries. However, now I like to do Bikram yoga with twenty or thirty other people, all struggling and sweating profusely. Though his pictures showed his body in great shape, it was his facial transformation that drew my attention. Here was a man who knew how to make his face young again. I was ready to learn from him.

He insisted that the smoothness of his skin was due solely to persistent daily friction combined with exercises for the face, neck, and throat. His first secret to facial rejuvenation is friction. Sound familiar? I already knew this from my own experience. Bennett writes: "The true secret of restoring to the skin the smoothness of youth is friction. The skin can be polished and the wrinkles rubbed out like any other piece of leather, and the palms of the hands and the tips of the fingers are the very best tools to use for that purpose."

I quite agree with the importance of applying friction to the skin. I use the term *exfoliation*. Friction applied to the skin is exfoliation. I came to the idea of dry-brushing my face entirely on my own. I don't think the palms of the hands produce enough friction, however. Throughout his book, Bennett advocates using your dry palms. Mine are definitely not rough enough for adequate exfoliation. The facial brush I've designed is ideal for accomplishing the kind of friction that

Bennett advocates. Be sure to brush your face before going to bed.

Keep up your twice a day facial exercise routine.

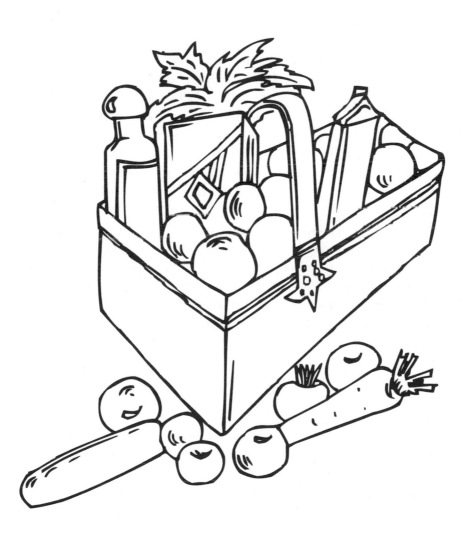

Day 19

Bennett's second secret to facial rejuvenation is muscle stimulation. Muscles, he reminds us, are augmented by alternating contraction and relaxation, or by deep tissue massage. The increased blood flow caused by such actions burns carbon, trims fat, and expels toxins.

To understand his approach and make the most of it, it is important to distinguish two basic types of muscles: voluntary and involuntary. Think in terms of active and passive, with active (voluntary) being those you can and do control, and passive (involuntary) as being those that motor along without your interference. As an example, you can wiggle your fingers at will, but your heart does its thing without any input from you. Your subconscious brain is in control of such muscles. Remembering to breathe and execute heartbeats would be just *too* much! Muscles in our arms, legs, fingers, toes, etc. are under conscious control and are, therefore, voluntary.

Bennett's system comes down to this: All facial muscles must be deep-massaged every day. He believed that gentle, superficial facial massage is good for conditioning the skin, but inadequate for developing supporting muscles. He suggested that speedy enlargement of the muscles could take place if they are *deeply* massaged. They must be rubbed firmly and systematically to make the change permanent.

Bennett based his theories of exercise on the practices of C.A. Sampson, one of the world's strongest men, who fastened strong elastic bands or straps tightly around his arms during dumb-bell exercises. The alternate pressure and relaxation of the bands made for a very effective massage. Sampson attributed his marvelous muscle development to this practice.

Bennett suggests that we contract voluntary muscles to greatly improve results. When muscles are contracted and vigorously massaged with the palms of the hands, he says, they quickly respond. I want to draw your attention to the word *contracted*. If you contract the muscles, then vigorously massage them, this will make a big difference in how your muscles respond. All voluntary muscles must be exercised with deep massaging applied at the same time.

From this day forward, add exercise 16 to your twice a day facial exercise routine.

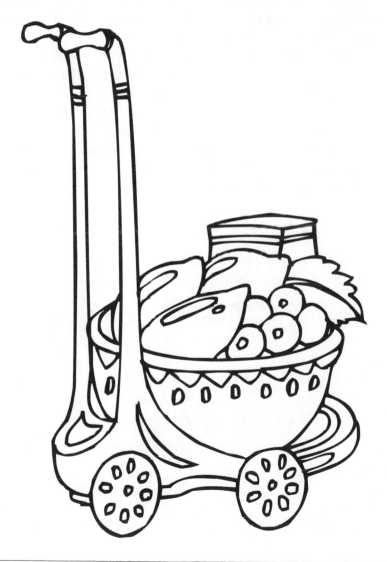

Day 20

Deep massage is especially effective when applied to the facial cheek muscles, perhaps because they typically have not been stimulated by exercise. When we're young, the muscles are strong and elastic; they support the tissue and skin overlying them, giving cheeks the full, round appearance characteristic of youth. There are eight long muscles, four on each side of the face. They are attached to the wide muscular band surrounding the mouth. As we age, they provide no adequate support, and the skin that covers them falls into creases and lines. Cheeks sink in and hollows appear because the supporting muscles have collapsed.

Bennett writes: "I do not claim that large muscles produced by this method indicate great strength, but as a means of speedily filling up the cheeks, rounding out the chin and the muscles covering the jaws, no other method yet devised will at all compare to it in efficiency."

Try this recipe today:

Cucumber Delight

In the morning juice:

3 cucumbers

1/2 a stalk of celery

1/4 onion

1 red pepper

1/2 a peeled lemon

Refrigerate approximately 1 cup and drink the remaining juice.

For your lunch, combine in a blender:

Leftover juice

1 avocado

handful of fresh cilantro

dash of garlic

dash of Celtic sea salt

Pour into bowl and sprinkle with:

fresh or dried dill

chopped scallions

additional chopped cucumber

Keep up your twice a day facial exercise routine.

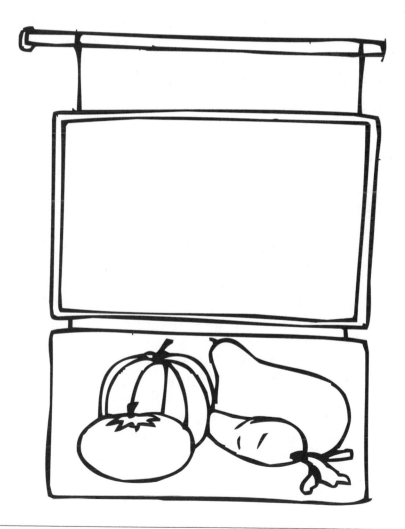

Day 21

All muscles have the same property: they grow when they're exercised and when they're not, they shrink. Moreover, they lose their strength and elasticity. What's the message? To get results, you must massage *daily* for at least a few minutes. Going for a deep tissue massage once per month, or even once a week, is not enough. Perform your facial massage daily. No more than one day off a week.

Newcomers always feel more improvement in the early stages of training. It's a fact—sluggish, involuntary muscles do respond more quickly to vigorous massage than do muscles accustomed to external stress like big muscles of the chest, arms, and legs. This massaging provides cross-fiber friction that effectively reduces adhesions (stuck tissue) and varying degrees of scar tissue formation in the soft tissues. This allows for a true freeing of tissues. The texture of the skin improves with the exercises. Stimulating your facial muscles will help metabolize fat deposits and retained water. If you perform facial exercises together with deep massaging, the combination will greatly improve circulation and rejuvenate your skin.

Our friend Bennett believed that daily palm massages strengthened facial capillaries. Be careful not to chafe the skin or make your muscles sore. Bennett starts with twenty strokes and builds up gradually. Pace yourself. You *train* for a marathon—you don't just run it. Go *gently*. But be persistent.

Don't dismiss massaging techniques for fear you will develop a broken capillary. Please realize that only weakened capillaries can be broken. If you are not eating a lot of raw fruits and vegetables foods, you will be at greater risk. You will be missing out, not taking advantage of the single most powerful anti-aging technique ever known. You must strengthen your skin tissues *from the inside* to protect them from becoming so fragile. If we want to look good in our mature years, raw foods is *definitely* the way to go. I greatly improved my appearance following the raw foods lifestyle and you can do the same. Read my books *Your Right to Be Beautiful* and *Beautiful on Raw* for more information.

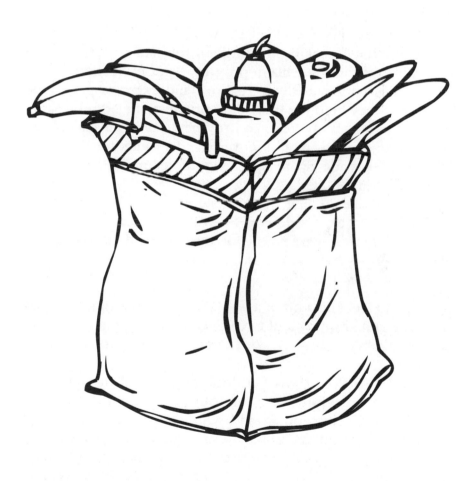

Take your "After" pictures. If you are happy with your results send me your "before" and "after" pictures, so others can be encouraged by your progress.

ATTENTION

Not-So Last Word

Sorry!

There just plain isn't a last word. It's all about getting better. As you'll hear in meetings of the famous twelve-step recovery program, "we claim progress—not perfection."

So it is with nutritional regimes and exercise programs: insofar as they help the individual progress, they do the same for the authors. I'm already on my next book. I'll make revisions to this one as new discoveries arise, whether these discoveries are made by me, the scientific community, or other innovators in the field.

And I'll keep doing these facial exercises, and try variations on them. So should you. Be willing, please, to be and to feel *awkward*. A wise friend of mine is fond of saying: *All learning is awkward. And all awkwardness is learning—if you know how to use it.*

So you feel like a bit of a goof, sitting there grimacing and wincing and grinning and tweaking and rubbing and making funny rubber faces as you exercise and massage…Get over it!

What?—Do you think you look magnificent in your aerobics class or while working out at the gym? Imagine someone following you around with a "fanny-cam," capturing your least elegant moments from your least advantageous perspective. You won't watch the results on playback more than once. But you'll be glad you exercised or lifted weights or pretzeled yourself at yoga class. It's the *results* that count.

And the progress. Precision counts toward that progress you want to realize day by day, week by week. So follow instructions, please, before you depart, vary or adapt. *Then* innovate. Regularity counts. Stick to your schedule. And have a sense of humor, will you? The kids will say, if they catch you facial-exercising: *Mommy looks funny.* Daddy will agree: *Mommy looks like a moron.* Well, you can laugh at them as they mimic you. And laugh at yourself, too. One of the biggest keys to progress, I believe, is taking things seriously. But never *too* seriously.

Don't take aging seriously. Think about it: we can look 10 years younger just by making funny faces. I'm *determined* to exercise my face—like the rest of my body—for all of my life, and I hope you will too.

May you enjoy a Rawsome Life and reveal your Rawsome Beauty!

Best wishes for your success!

Tonya Zavasta

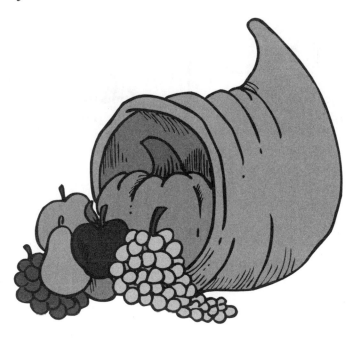

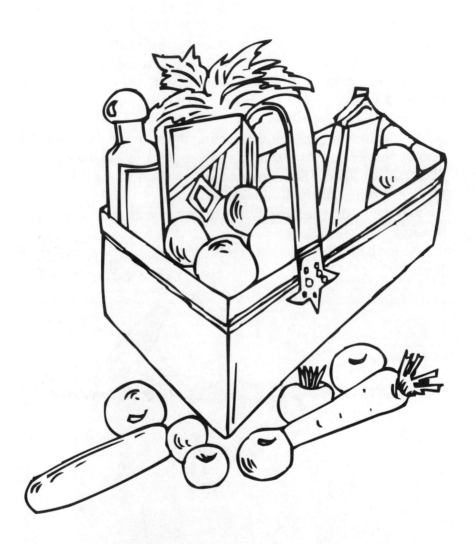

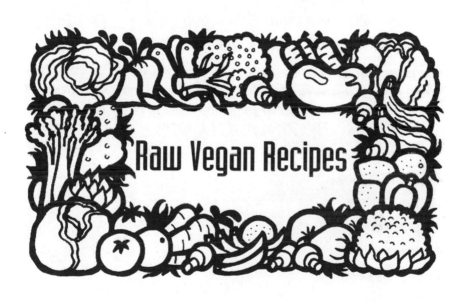

Raw Vegan Recipes

Raw Chili Bowl

1 cup chopped fresh tomatoes

½ cup sundried tomatoes, soaked for a few hours

1 cup chopped zucchini

1 clove garlic

2 TBS diced sweet onion

2 TBS chili powder

1 TBS cumin powder

¼ tsp cloves or cinnamon

dash of raw honey or agave nectar

Combine all the ingredients in a blender. In a separate large bowl combine 1 cup of chopped fresh tomatoes, 1 chopped avocado and red pepper to taste. Pour the blended mixture over the chopped tomatoes and avocado. Serves 2

Crudite Dream

Veggie Platter:

1 zucchini

1 tomato

1 red bell pepper

1 cucumber

Sauce:

½ cup coconut water

¼ cup macadamia nuts

¼ cup cashews or pine nuts

several fresh mint leaves

Slice all the Veggie Platter ingredients very thinly and arrange attractively on a colorful platter. Blend the Sauce ingredients thoroughly in a blender until smooth; drizzle the Sauce over the vegetables on the platter and garnish with mint leaves and nasturtium flowers. Serves 2

Peach Pudding Supreme

In a blender or food processor combine the following and blend until completely smooth:

2 fresh peaches

1 fresh or frozen banana

½ avocado

1TBS soaked chia seed

Pour the pudding into a bowl and eat with a spoon and a smile.

Serves 1

Creamy Tomato Soup

This quick and easy soup serves 2

4 chopped fresh tomatoes

1 cup water

¼ cup chopped onion

½ cup raw tahini (or pine nuts)

small handful of fresh basil

Blend all until smooth and garnish with fresh basil and a sprinkle of dulse flakes.

Stuffed Red Peppers

4-5 ripe red or orange bell peppers

½ cup chopped tomato

½ cup sundried tomatoes, soaked

¼ cup each of chopped carrot and celery

½ cup of soaked walnuts

¼ *cup chopped apple*

2 TBS fresh lemon juice

fresh thyme to taste

Slice the tops off of the peppers and scoop out the insides. Blend the remaining ingredients in a blender or food processor and then scoop out and stuff into the peppers. Garnish with fresh thyme and parsley.

Serves 2

Pear Up Salad

2 cups of fresh spinach or other greens of your choice

2 fresh pears, chopped

1 stalk celery, diced

½ *cup raisins*

½ *cup walnuts, chopped*

juice from 1 orange

Arrange greens on a serving plate. Toss together the remaining ingredients and serve on top of the greens for a very simple and delicious salad.

Serves 1-2

Summer Salsa

2 cups diced tomatoes

¼ *onion, diced*

½ *yellow bell pepper, diced*

½ *orange bell pepper, diced*

1 jalapeno, de-seeded and diced

½ *cup fresh cilantro, chopped*

1 clove garlic, finely diced

juice of 1 lime

pinch of sea salt (optional)

1 avocado, chopped (optional)

Combine thoroughly in a mixing bowl and serve with vegetable crudités. Thinly sliced jicama tastes especially good.

Serves 2

Eggplant Toss

Peel and dice one eggplant and 2 avocados. Combine in a serving bowl with the juice of 1 lemon and enough water to barely cover. Leave to soak while you whisk together a dressing in a small bowl using the following:

2 TBS olive oil

1 clove chopped garlic

2 TBS chopped onion

two pinches of dulse flakes, more if desired

juice of 1 lemon

Drain the eggplant and avocado thoroughly to remove the bitterness. Toss with the dressing and leave in the refrigerator for 15–30 minutes to marinade before serving.

Serves 2

Blackberry Parfait

2 cups of fresh blackberries

1 sliced banana

1 cup raisins

½ cup chopped soaked almonds or other soaked nuts

Place the blackberries in a pretty bowl (preferably a deep one) and layer with the other ingredients in any order you prefer.

Top with a generous dollop of almond butter and a dusting of cinnamon

Drizzle with either agave syrup or honey (optional)

Serves 1-2

Handful Salad

Toss together in a bowl:

2 big handfuls of fresh broccoli, chopped

a handful of golden raisins

a handful of soaked sunflower seeds

two pinches of chopped onion

For the dressing, whisk together the following in a small bowl:

3 TBS almond butter

2 TBS agave nectar or raw honey

enough water to achieve the desired consistency

Toss the dressing with the salad.

Serves 1-2

Soup's On!

Cream of Cauliflower

Juice approximately 7 carrots and 1 inch of ginger root in the morning, or enough to drink for breakfast and reserve 2 cups of juice for later. At lunchtime, combine the following ingredients in a blender and blend until smooth:

2 cups remaining carrot/ginger juice (or you could use 1 cup juice and 1 cup almond milk)

1 cup cauliflower

1 avocado

1 TSP each of garam masala and curry powder

Garnish with diced red pepper, chopped cauliflower or some crumbled dried nori if you like. Serves 1-2

Simple Borscht

In the morning, juice 2 medium beets, 6 or 7 stalks of celery and 8 carrots, or enough to drink for breakfast and reserve 2 cups of juice for later. At lunchtime, combine in a bowl the 2 cups of leftover juice, ½ freshly juiced lemon (or orange if you prefer), a pinch of garlic and a pinch of sea salt. Top with fresh dill and ½ diced avocado, along with a little grated beet. Adding a few spoonfuls of raw saurkraut is lovely too. Serves 1-2

Corn Chowder (Oh, how I love this soup!)

Juice approximately 8 carrots, 6 celery stalks, 2 leeks and a handful of parsley, or enough to drink for breakfast and reserve 2 cups of juice for later. At lunchtime, combine the following ingredients in a blender:

2 cups remaining morning juice

1 avocado

1 cup of raw corn kernels cut from the cob

1 TSP coconut oil

a pinch of sea salt

Blend until smooth and garnish with more fresh corn kernels and chopped parsley and dust with herbs such as thyme or marjoram. Serves 1-2

Hemp Sprinkle

Juice approximately 3 carrots, a handful of spinach, 2 stalks of celery and a peeled orange, or enough to drink for breakfast and have 2 cups left over for later. At lunchtime, grate some carrots in a bowl, add a few sprigs of fresh (not dried) rosemary or sage, and pour the remaining 2 cups of morning juice on top. Sprinkle with a generous handful of hemp seeds and a crumbled sheet of nori. Serves 1-2

Dynamic Duo

A match made in heaven!

This recipe uses 'Scarlet Beauty Juice' from Beautiful on Raw: Uncooked Creations *as a base for 'Victoria's Favorite' from her* Green for Life.

Juice approximately 5 tomatoes, 2 carrots and 1 medium beet for your morning juice but save 1 cup for the lunchtime soup. At lunchtime, combine the following in a blender:

1 cup remaining morning juice

6 leaves red lettuce

¼ bunch basil

juice of ½ lime

¼ red onion

2 celery stalks

¼ avocado

Blend until smooth and pour into a bowl over a crumbled nori sheet and a few sundried tomatoes. Top with a handful of pine nuts. Serves 1-2

Asparagus Carrot

Make plain carrot juice in the morning, enough to drink and save 1 cup for later. At lunchtime, combine the following in a blender:

1 cup remaining morning juice

1 cup chopped asparagus

2 TBS tahini or almond butter

1-2 TSP of diced onion

Blend until smooth and pour into bowl. Top with extra chopped asparagus and one of the following to taste: sea salt, chopped nori or Bragg's dulse flakes. Serves 1-2